CW01064303

Transplants and Fears

Christopher Simpson

Grosvenor House
Publishing Limited

All rights reserved
Copyright © Christopher Simpson, 2023

The right of Christopher Simpson to be identified as the author of this
work has been asserted in accordance with Section 78
of the Copyright, Designs and Patents Act 1988

The book cover is copyright to Christopher Simpson

This book is published by
Grosvenor House Publishing Ltd
Link House
140 The Broadway, Tolworth, Surrey, KT6 7HT.
www.grosvenorhousepublishing.co.uk

This book is sold subject to the conditions that it shall not, by way of
trade or otherwise, be lent, resold, hired out or otherwise circulated
without the author's or publisher's prior consent in any form of binding or
cover other than that in which it is published and
without a similar condition including this condition being imposed
on the subsequent purchaser.

A CIP record for this book
is available from the British Library

ISBN 978-1-80381-453-7

Transplants and Fears

The courageous story of Christopher Michael Simpson

Co Wrote by

Bee Ross

A true story about a boy growing up in the world of medical interventions and kidney transplants. Using true grit, determination and humour to survive his ordeals, his inspirational journey is an account of mental health challenges and relationship difficulties, and it has all the thrills and spills of a Hollywood blockbuster.

This account is written with the down-to-earth reality of lived experience that any patient can relate to, and from which any health or social care professional can learn.

Special Thanks to Mum

Contents

Foreword

For over thirty years, Chris has experienced the highs and lows of kidney disease – from successful kidney transplantation to its subsequent failure and a return to dialysis. Throughout this time, he has been determined to live as normal a life as possible.

This book is the emotional and honest journey of a young man living with kidney disease. I am sure it will be a great help to other patients, their relatives and those who care for them in understanding the life-altering effect of kidney failure and, more importantly, how to survive this.

– Dr Stuart Robertson, Consultant Nephrologist, Wrexham Maelor Hospital

Introduction

Hi All,

I am Christopher, the author of this life story.

I am, the only child of Wendy and Kevin, a working-class family from Manchester in the mid-1980's. Mother and Father's relationship took a strain and after two years they finally went their separate ways and ended their relationship. My mother then went on to have another relationship, which gave me my sister Claire.

I grew up with many health complications which began when I was born prematurely. My young Mother and Father had to make many impossible decisions about my care. My life can only be explained as a blend of medical marvels and true grit and determination on the part of myself and my family.

Having dealt with the complexities of kidney failure and numerous transplants, I learnt more than most to appreciate life and live for each day because tomorrows are never promised. I grew up on a council estate in the thriving city of Manchester UK. Due to my extensive hospital stays and interventions, I did not achieve the highest education, though I did miraculously attain my GCSEs to a good enough standard. More than education, my passion to help others grew and by showing courage and resilience against the odds I feel that I have achieved what most people can only dream of.

Many of you may be wondering what it was that made me embark on writing a book about my life with kidney failure, and thus shedding light on the very real, though relatable, struggles with my mental health.

I originally started to write some things down that came to mind from the age of about 19 years old. However, I quickly lost concentration. I am sure you will come to appreciate this while reading through my life's journey. I had a lot to contend with, including whether I believe that my life journey was good enough to share with others. In my head, I thought: what good could come of this if I was to open my heart for everyone else to see? To make judgements on the decisions that I have to make, or others have had to make on my behalf.

I always had the ambition and passion to help and support others. I have always had the vision of hope that I could provide an understanding of the hidden side effects suffered by an individual and their family when living with such a chronic life-changing condition. The one thing I lack is confidence and knowing where to start.

It was while working with Caron, my amazing social worker who helped me restore my confidence and break down barriers, that my life took a turn for the better. Even when I knew, and soon so will you, that all good things come to an end. Especially in my life! But you can read about these events in this book. Caron introduced me to a lady called Elizabeth Lefroy, or Liz for short. Liz is the programme leader of a Social Work degree course at Wrexham's Glyndŵr University. Liz and Caron had previously discussed the benefit to me of being part of a 'service users' group called Outside In.

The Outside In members are made up of all age ranges with many different health and social care needs. The idea of the group is to support and add further teaching and perspective for Social Work students. This helps the students, along with the teaching staff, to get a better understanding of the complexities faced by health and social care staff when working with individuals within that sector. Some of the Outside In members, who are an amazing group of individuals, have a wide range of needs. Some have hidden needs while some of the individuals have quite visible needs.

Communication is the biggest factor in the group and by helping to break down barriers between students and individuals it is hoped that the level of care and compassion goes further, in order to make all health and social care diverse and best fit for the individuals accessing the help and support. These aims are achieved through sharing our lived experiences of having Social Services and health support in our lives and how effective they have or have not been. The aim is to teach students how to positively communicate through real-life conflicts good or bad. All that is shared between the group and the students is always confidential. This has allowed me the space to realise that in joining this Outside In group I was able to achieve my vision of help and support, even if it was in a completely different way than I had imagined.

After a week of introductions and a settling in period, I was put into a small group. The aim of the group was to forge some initial alliances and to alleviate any discomforts I may have been feeling. Each Outside In member was allocated a small group of around 4 or 5 social work students. This was how I met Bee, Rhi, Hannah and Hayley. When they were asking questions, I panicked a little instead of explaining my condition or how I came to join the group. I blurted out that I had been writing about my life story. They were all full of encouragement and helped me to see the potential my story could bring in helping others. Bee was quick to point out that my story had the potential to help patients going through similar conditions, and that it could also assist in the education of new students and medical professionals.

After some exceptional guidance from Liz, the tutor, and the surprisingly quick but mutual friendship that had developed between myself and Bee, I began to see a future in my idea of writing such a personal book. Hopefully this will leave a lasting legacy well after I am no longer here.

It was at the start of the Covid-19 pandemic, when the world was fragile with uncertainties and fear, that Bee came up with an ingenious idea. She had the idea of producing a draft copy of an entire book. Her view was that if we managed to produce a draft of a book with all my ideas in, I would have a positive achievement to look back on, even if it stayed on my own bookshelves.

So, we decided to have a go at bringing my dream to life. Bee knew even in such a short space of time that my dreams of helping others are very important to me. Miraculously we made a commitment to this project. To now see the achievement and progress is an unimaginable and heart-warming experience. This book is our collaboration and proof that through hard work, commitment and determination sprinkled with true friendship, results and dreams really can come true.

During the lockdown, Caron introduced me, Bee and Liz, to a considerate, empathetic and passionate lady called Judith. Judith was the Managing Director of Kidney Wales, and through our many meetings, we all worked towards one goal. Judith and Caron both took the rough draft and read it through.

Liz had the idea to possibly get my lived experience on to Health and Social Care university recommended reading lists, in the hope of further spreading awareness of the hidden disabilities and complexities of Chronic Kidney Disease (CKD). As part of my commitment to Glyndŵr and the Outside In group, I agreed to have a few copies of the book in the library to help promote awareness of the Outside In group project. It is thought that the collaboration of the different agencies would promote the elite and exceptional learning opportunities of Glyndŵr's BA (Hons) undergraduate Social Work programme for students and other agencies involved in delivering the course. Students affiliated with Glyndŵr acquire the outstanding unrivalled experience and knowledge learnt from individuals who have shared their lived experiences via the Outside In group. This has reaped far more rewards than can ever be gained from textbooks.

My future hope is that in some way my book will give a real-life witness to common, yet devastating, battles fought by many that go unnoticed. This will raise awareness of the complexities of physical illness such has CKD and mental illness, stressing the importance of giving individuals or patients autonomy in their life decisions. The book will shed light on some of the previously unspoken situations dealt with in families, when a child or young person has to deal with many changing situations. My aim for the book is to bring a true, non-filtered look into the way a patient or service user is seen and heard in life, and to reveal the effectiveness that practitioners can have upon the life of the individuals for whom they provide care and support. I hope that future generations of professionals take into consideration the impact that each decision and action can have.

I hope you are well and that you will be able to see how personal this book is to me, and that my hopes and dreams are to some extent being achieved. Keep pushing yourself to the next goal. Ask for help when you feel low or lonely, but most of all treat others how you would want to be treated. You never know when life could take a devasting or life-changing twist.

Stay safe and healthy,

Christopher

CHAPTER 1
Birth and Diagnosis

Some people struggle with normal things in life such as getting to work on time, holding down a job, or even finding the right life partner. What if I were to tell you I would give the world for these struggles? Do not get me wrong, I'm not disregarding the difficulties, or that others have different opinions and views on situations, but I sit alone most of the time wondering...what would it be like to be normal?

Maybe I should take you on a journey through my life one step at a time.

Buckle up and sit back, make sure you're comfortable, oh, and stock up on all the things that get you through the tough times in life, the sadness, the disappointment, the anger, the frustration, and of course, those things which support you in celebrating the good times: the achievements, the laughter and the proudest of moments. For me, I hold tight to friends, family, and some other inspirational characters I have met along my journey. This is a journey of a baby born prematurely, not only fighting to survive but fighting against his own body.

I must add here that I have a wicked sense of humour: after all, at times that is the only thing that has kept my fight alive. Oh, and a few medical interventions, medical staff, machines, procedures, drugs, the list goes on.

Are you comfortable? Then let us begin.

Wendy, my Mum, speaks

Rushed down a long narrow hospital corridor not knowing what to expect at twenty-one years old. The first time – I'm in so much pain. Is this it? Am I in labour? Surely, I can't be. I'm only 28 weeks. Surely this isn't the baby coming? But I believe it is.

A cold, pale corridor with long strips of bright light...large fingerprint covered windows and grey-blue nonslip floors with a yellow handrail that spans for what feels like miles... people standing in alcoves scantily draped in gowns, hiding their modesty, well almost. The odd glance of veins decorating a bare leg and fashionable new slippers.

Doctors and nurses walking briskly towards their mission to serve the sick and needy while controlling the onslaught of visitors.

The pains are shooting from one side of my swelling tummy and along my back. My breath is short and desperate.

The wheelchair in which I sit gives the most uncomfortable position of all. My heart is racing but not as quickly as the thoughts penetrating my mind. The scariest thoughts and desperation in my voice...an observant nurse looks and in an instant I'm taken behind a busy-patterned curtain. This causes a stirring of commotion amongst the staff.

This is where Chris's story began.

Day-by-day I walk along these long cold and lonely corridors with the constant conveyor belt of expectant mothers in wheelchairs, and onlookers, visitors of new mothers, proud grandparents, and excited fathers. I catch glimpses of healthy babies born wide-eyed with the world at their disposal, a sense of wonder dancing across their tiny perfectly formed faces, their families glowing with pride and anxiety, excitement and fear mixed in equal measure, and the realisation that these bundles of joy are going to be depending on them for every lifeline.

These tiny infants are blessed with the security of family and friends, but more importantly, with their health and an abundance of love and protection. Though, all I can think of at this moment is my premature baby, all alone, struggling to survive, his body weak from exhaustion, trying to recover from the experience of a birth that occurred far too early.

I have spent almost a week now in this hospital ward, feeling like a failure and a fraud. My baby is nowhere to be seen, yet my body knows it has been through the trauma of childbirth, the ordeal of premature birth with extreme complications. All these thoughts and feelings are swirling around my brain. Without my baby by my side.

The first few weeks of his life. Instead, I have an empty chair prepared for visitors placed next to my bed.

Talking about my bed, that itself should almost certainly come with a warning. The hard-base mattress is balanced on the hardness of the rails. It is finished with a bright white sheet and the most uncomfortable pillow with matching pillowcase, all with army-style tightly tucked edges, topped with another white sheet and a circular blanket that causes my skin to itch. The blanket is a sage green with the name of the hospital sewn into it. All beds uniformed to a specific colour for each of the wards.

The ward has seven hospital beds, each separated by bizarrely decorated curtains, which the staff pull around the confinements of each bed, thinking this gives privacy. Yet everyone around can listen to the most personal of conversations, regardless of the nurses' intentions, there's no privacy here.

The ward I was occupying was full: the other six new mums had their babies next to their beds most of the day.

The regular chorus of infant song would pour around the walls and fill the corridors linking the ward to the nurses' station. These sounds could be heard from outside the infant nursery room too. Yet my baby was nowhere to be seen. I witnessed the confused glances from the other women and their visitors when they looked over expectantly towards my space.

Consumed with anxiety and fear-stricken thoughts, I decided to close my curtains permanently, only leaving a gap big enough for me to gaze out of the window from time to time, and watch the birds tapping their feet while whistling beautiful melodies. It was whilst watching these birds that I decided that when Kevin (the baby's father) came to visit, we should decide on a name for our precious baby boy.

We should bring his existence to life and honour him with a name after all. He had endured so much in such a short space of time - this baby boy's fight was strong.

For such a tiny, poorly baby he was showing real strength and determination to be alive. True to my word, when Kevin came to visit, we decided on a name.

Our boy Is now called Christopher Michael Simpson. A strong name for such a strong boy. Christopher was now a week old, however, he was still extremely small and fragile. I remember as I looked in on him in his warm incubator, he looked so peaceful and settled. At the same time, I was witnessing all the assistance of the incubator. A heat mat to regulate his temperature. The narrow tubes poking from between his ribs draining his chest and allowing his breathing to be free and less consuming of his energy. Then there were the tubes forced down his cute button nose directly into his abdomen and taped securely to his cheek.

I'm so grateful to all medical staff and I could never repay them for their compassion and care, but at this moment I felt sad. I'd always wanted to breastfeed my baby, to feel the closeness and the unconditional loving bond between mother and baby. For me, the best I was going to get was to express my milk for the nurses to prepare for Christopher. Fortunately though, I was over-producing milk. One of the special care nurses suggested that I express my milk to help the other poorly babies. So, this is what I did. It gave me a sense of purpose, which I would have struggled to find otherwise.

Christopher was transferred to Pendlebury Children's Hospital when he was thirty hours old. Kevin and I were sat watching over Christopher like the terrified parents we were. I would stop over with Christopher while Kevin usually came after work in the evening.

I think it was roughly within the first 24 hours that we were told, by a specialist, that Christopher had been born with Bladder Outlet Obstruction.

This occurs when the urethra, the tube that carries urine from the bladder out of the body, is too narrow or blocked. This blockage causes urine to back up in the bladder, placing an unborn baby at risk of kidney and lung problems. Bladder Outlet Obstruction is also known as Foetal Lower Urinary Tract Obstruction (LUTO).

Christopher was also confirmed by the specialist to have Posterior Urethral Valves (PUV's) also referred to as Congenital Obstructing Posterior Urethral Membranes or COPUM for short. PUV is an obstructive developmental anomaly in the urethra and genital-urinary system of male new-borns.

A posterior urethral valve is an obstructing membrane in the posterior male urethra as a result of abnormal in-utero development. It is the most common cause of bladder outlet obstruction in male new-borns.

PUV varies in degree, with mild cases presenting late due to reduced symptoms. Babies affected more severely can have renal and respiratory failure from lung underdevelopment as a result of low amniotic fluid volumes, requiring intensive care and close monitoring. It occurs in about one in 8000 babies. There has been more recent research that concludes that PUV can also be hereditary. This was not the case in our family.

It was becoming apparent that Christopher was suffering from a severe case of PUV, but had the specialist confirmed that Christopher's kidneys and bladder were not working efficiently? If he had, this should have prepared me for what was going to follow.

The medical team that was overseeing Christopher's care had all decided on setting a reasonable target weight for Christopher to attain. By the age of 2 weeks, Christopher was having his chest drains removed. This was a huge step in the right direction and could only be a positive leap in Christopher's development. The nursing staff explained that Christopher was now able to breathe of his own accord.

The past two weeks had been long and arduous, but all the moments of sadness and worry were being washed away by the new feelings. I looked down into Christopher's blue eyes and saw him studying my face.

I stroked my shaking fingers down his small but swollen cheeks and felt the smooth downy hairs along his face and neck. His skin was almost translucent, but warm. His chest was rising and falling rhythmically – this calmed my soul and soothed my nervous breath.

The tears flowed from my eyes, rolled down my nose, and created droplets of pure love on Christopher's tummy. My boy: so small and so mighty – still attached to numerous tubes for feeding and antibiotics. Nevertheless, he was finally in my arms.

The overwhelming sense caught between our mutual gaze was that we would be there for each other, fighting battles and winning them a step at a time.

I was constantly reminded by the hospital staff that this was going to be a long journey, and each day would bring challenges and changes to which we must adapt.

Christopher is now one-month old and is starting to put on the required weight, but unfortunately, my baby boy is in a lot of pain and discomfort.

He is unable to stabilise his temperature and is getting frequent infections. Christopher's specialist was asking colleagues from other hospitals for reassurance and second opinions, making sure that Christopher was getting the best treatment and interventions available to him. A bladder specialist (also known as a Nephrologist) joined his medical team.

The Nephrologist explained that Christopher's bladder was not working correctly and that performing a procedure on his urethra might help the issues with his kidneys. This procedure, called a vesicostomy, is an opening created by the doctor between the abdominal wall and the bladder. This helps prevent harm to the kidneys. This surgery is done in the operating room. The opening looks like a small slit with pink tissue all around it. Urine drains constantly from this opening, and the child will need to wear a diaper, pull-ups, or an incontinence pad, such as Poise Pads. A vesicostomy is a temporary treatment.

This surgery is a necessary step for some children to help prevent urinary tract infections and/or harm to the kidney. Most children who need a vesicostomy are young (under 5 years old) but sometimes older children or teenagers need this surgery temporarily.

At only a month old, my baby has already been through so much pain and suffering and is now going to endure surgery. I struggle with the very thought of my baby boy, so extraordinarily little and vulnerable, having to go to the theatre for such invasive surgery. Then I am told that this procedure is going to be the first of many surgeries that my infant is going to require. I feel sick to the stomach with worry. My head spins with images: all the things that I may never get to experience with my brave boy, and thoughts of Christopher lying in theatre with surgeons cutting into his tiny body.

The Nephrologist reminds me that without this procedure Christopher would unquestionably suffer further complications with fatal consequences.

The decision is made for me, and I give consent for my baby to undergo this procedure. I kiss my baby for what could be the last time. Christopher seems settled and calm: he is such a good boy. The nurse returns with the forms and with a shaky hand I sign the paperwork, tears yet again filling my eyes.

I wholeheartedly trust the specialist but this boy, my brave boy, is my boy. The baby I vowed to care for, the baby I carried inside my body, close to my heart. The baby that kicked me and kept me awake so many nights. My unrelenting love spills from my very veins for this boy. With this fleeting thought, I catch sight of the theatre team and from the window I see a brief meeting taking place between staff members discussing the plan. The surgeon pops into the bay. I stand holding Christopher's hand through the circular flaps of his incubator.

He looks me in the eye with a gentle smile and says we are ready now.

The tears roll from my eyes. I kiss my index and middle fingers and lay them upon my brave boy's chest. I step back and two nurses wheel my boy through soft-closing double doors. The wait begins and the anxiety fills the space between my heart and my head in Kevin's arms as he squeezes my hand to reassure me. But all I want is the sound of those soft-closing doors to open and the words from the theatre staff that Christopher is in recovery and doing well.

The minutes pass slowly, so do the hours. Time seems to have stopped. Corridors are quieter than normal. The sounds of the ward retreats. But the ticks of the clock are loud. I can feel my heart racing and my pulse quickening.

My eyes become heavy. I drift off to sleep. The sleep feels short, but two hours later I'm woken by Kevin tapping hurriedly on my shoulder.

My baby lies in his cot, now not needing an incubator, dressed in a clean nappy and a woollen bonnet. The nurse smiles at me and says I can look at my boy but must refrain from touching him until the surgeon can give me an update. Christopher has been given medicine to keep his pain to a minimum, but she warns he may become restless and upset due to the anaesthetic.

I take a deep cleansing breath, move towards Christopher's space. I feel so elated to have my brave boy back but frustrated that I can't hold him.

The feelings running through my head then can only be described as excitement and nervousness. I was finally able to hold my baby son in my arms for the very first time.

It was March 9th, Mothers' Day!

CHAPTER 2
Kidney Transplant 1

After many weeks of tests and doctors prodding and poking at my fearless baby boy, Christopher's consultant sauntered on to the ward with a look on his face with which I was unfamiliar.

He put his expert hand gently but firmly on mine, and looked straight into my eyes, demanding all my attention, and boy did he have it, especially when he muttered the words, "I have news". At that moment my heart dropped to the floor, the rest of my body feeling like it was going to follow. My eyes instantly filled with the tears that had been waiting to emerge all day.

It was as if my motherly instincts kicked in – they felt like a knot in my tummy. I grew used to these feelings, and at times they felt like the only things that I could rely on. Whether I wanted them or not, they kept me company.

In a split moment, the ever-busy ward, normally flooded with staff, babies, and visitors, became deafeningly still and calm. The consultant remarked, "Why the tears? It's good news!" He carried on talking, but my ears were not functioning. I remember looking for a seat to flop on, to support my weight. I then said hurriedly, "Can you repeat your words, please? I thought for a moment you said it was good news."

He smiled widely and let go of my hands. He had another check over Christopher's records.

Then he explained. "Do you recall that around six weeks ago, as Christopher's specialist medical team, we all agreed that his target weight should be set at around 5lbs?" I nodded, still unsure of my understanding.

He carried on: "Earlier this morning, we gave Christopher a thorough once over, his weight being 5lb 1oz, and taking into consideration his excellent progress, we believe as a team that this might be a fantastic opportunity for Christopher to meet your friends and family and for you all to be able to go home together."

I started to cry again: this time the tears flowed so quickly that before I knew it, my top began to dampen. I squirmed in my seat with pure elation. I was so excited and nervous, but more than that I was thankful to this team of fantastic people.

The staff at the hospital had quickly become my family. They were there for me just as much as they were for Christopher. They never sighed at my questions, even though I asked the same question to each one, in turn, to try to get a better answer, or one that I would believe. Not once did they make me feel unimportant, nor did they tell me that it was my fault that Christopher was suffering like he was. Instead, they took their time to explain again and again until they were sure I fully understood what was happening and the reasons for that action being taken. They held my hand when I got scared, and they reminded me to take a break for food or a drink. They also made me giggle when they helped me to change Christopher's nappy and I put it on the wrong way, or when I would pronounce a doctor's name incorrectly.

Through all this, the staff – from the cleaners to the nurses, from the woman serving me in the shop to the consultants – were amazing. As a result, I could not help feeling a little apprehensive being told I could take my brave boy home without their support.

Just Kevin and me doing the care and feeds, the nappy changes, the medication, the constant temperature checks, and infection control. How was this going to unfold? My precious, brave baby son finally coming home.

Not knowing who to call first or tell, I just gazed in amazement over towards Christopher. I stood up and walked towards the cot and took his tiny fingers and said: "You're coming home with Mummy, my brave baby boy. You've done it. You're coming home!"

I looked up at the consultant and asked, "When can I take my baby home?"

His answer was crisp and clear: "All being well, tomorrow. We have already discussed follow-up appointments and medication. You have completed the training you need to continue with the tube feeding at home. So, to give you time to plan, let us say as long as Christopher continues to have a settled evening, we'll discharge him from the hospital by pre-lunchtime rounds tomorrow. I will plan for medication and further appointments with out-patients. If you've any questions, please ask. We are still here for you – you can phone at any time. I'll also arrange for a specialist midwife to contact you in the next few days." With that, he was gone.

With a cleansing breath my thoughts cleared, and I realised tomorrow would have been my expected due date. How special! I excitedly made for the door as Kevin walked in.

The words exploded from my mouth.

"He's coming home, we can take him home!" Kevin embraced me with the tightest cuddle: I could feel his heartbeat racing too. His first words were, "I'll go and get the car," but I quickly interjected, "Tomorrow, I mean he can come home tomorrow!" We both sat in absolute silence, not a word passed our lips, but a million thoughts were in our minds.

After Christopher was settled off to sleep for the evening at 6 pm, Kevin and I strolled along what had once felt like a long, narrow corridor. It was now full of colour and character. If walls could talk, I thought to myself, I wonder what these ones would say? After all, they have propped up the hysterical, and have witnessed excitement, along with the weeping sorrow of many. But our story is one of many twists and turns, and more emotions than I ever knew existed.

We went home that evening to prepare for Christopher's arrival. At first, I just stood staring at the floor space covered in baby items and washing. On every surface there were cards congratulating us on our new arrival. Yet they had been there so long that the dust had collected on them, and others had started to fade. I tossed off my boots and shrugged off my coat. Putting aside our belongings, I gave instructions to Kevin, asking him to shift all the stuff from the lounge and make the space ready for tomorrow when Christopher would be home with us after three long tiring months.

The next day came quicker than any other day. The light started to break through the net curtains, and the birds chirped in the bushes outside the window. Kevin was still snoring next to me like an elephant! I tiptoed downstairs and looked at all the necessities: piles of nappies, baby-grows, matching vests, and bottom cream. The changing mat leant across the sofa. Christopher was so small, still smaller than an average new-born. Tiny and fragile as he was, he was about to come home.

Once Christopher was safely home, I began to understand how life could now begin to take on the essence of normality, something that I'd only been able to imagine for the past few weeks.

Christopher lay in his bouncer chair content and happy, with his fingers moving in uncoordinated motions. His eyes twinkled when caught by the light and his nose was, still is, the cutest on the planet! I'm such a proud Mum, although I know I am over-protective, like a wild tiger with her cubs. I watched every breath that my baby took, and every flinch of his body.

Christopher was such a good baby, and he quickly settled into a routine. With check-up appointments and out-patient clinics, the days ticked by, and before we knew it, another momentous day had crept up on us.

Astonishingly, my brave baby boy survived to see his first birthday, something that we could never allow ourselves to imagine. Yet, there we were. We'd finally made it. In total disbelief, we were joined by both sets of grandparents to celebrate. Birthdays are a time for reflection as well as celebration, and we looked back over the past twelve months. What a rollercoaster we had all endured! However, this little boy makes every struggle worth it.

We were celebrating, but I was so scared of letting the moment pass without making a song and dance about it. Every breath I have taken since Christopher was born, I needed him a little closer to me - I can't stop holding him a little tighter every time I pick him up.

Even back then, on his first birthday, I realised I'd have to let him go at some point, especially when both grandmas were giving me that look. You know that look that says: when is it our time for cuddles? Can I have a hold of this miracle bundle of joy?

Christopher's determination and strong will power have seen him through all the tough times. Thankfully though, his birthday was his day to be celebrated. My special boy: one-year-old today! A day I'd never dared in my wildest dreams would come to pass.

The next year went on month by month. Slowly, but surely, Christopher's health started to deteriorate. We made the most of the good days and dealt with the bad days.

Christopher's happy-go-lucky character and his laidback charm kept us smiling on the fun days, and his sheer grit and determination spurred us on when the days were long and tough. The weather outside turned colder and the nights were getting longer. Christopher's immune system was failing, as his body struggled to cope under the pressure of his lacklustre kidney function.

The trees dropped their green foliage, their naked branches emptied of singing birds. The nearby homes brimmed with Christmas cheer, decorated with tinsel and fairy lights. Choruses of children sung hymns in the local church and robins graced our garden wall. But this was a Christmas to fear, as Christopher's health degenerated, and Christmas wishes became focused on just one: to keep my baby alive.

There were many appointments, blood tests, consultant reviews: most of all, Christopher's medication needed to be changed and reviewed. There were constant worries about what could be happening next. Then, in that December of 1987, came the phone call to beat all amazing calls: the answer to all our prayers, the one thing that surely would save my boy.

It came late on a bitterly cold, wet and windy evening: the piercing sound of the phone ringing in the night. It startled me from my sleep. Throwing on a dressing gown, I clambered down the stairs hoping the sound wouldn't wake Christopher, who had not long settled after a particularly tough and draining day for us both.

There was a voice on the other end of the phone that I instantly recognised: the sister from Wrigley Ward of Pendlebury Hospital, Salford, now known as the Royal Manchester Children's Hospital.

This new hospital had replaced services previously provided by the Pendlebury Children's Hospital in Salford, Booth Hall Children's Hospital at Blackley in north Manchester, and neonatal care from Saint Mary's Hospital, Manchester. The Royal is a combined hospital and was completed in June 2009.

The Sister explained that a match had become available for Christopher's kidney transplant. This transplant would save my boy's life. It would solve all his troubles, heal him from the pain and suffering. I was weeping as I asked the Sister to repeat her words and promise that this was not someone playing a joke.

After all, my boy's pain and fighting could and should stop as soon as he underwent this operation, for a long while at least.

The Sister explained with a sternness in her voice which demanded my full attention: "Gather Christopher's belongings and make your way to the hospital immediately. Time is of the essence and we do not want to pass this opportunity by." I replied, "Okay, we'll see you soon."

My heart was pounding, my palms were clammy, I felt a mix of delight and utter fear. I switched on the lights and made my way upstairs so quickly that I stumbled up them. It didn't matter that I bashed my shin - I burst into the bedroom and shook Kevin who was lying peacefully asleep. "Kevin, wake up, it's time: they have a match! We must get ready now and go to the hospital."

Kevin stirred, rubbing his eyes and recoiling at the light glaring bright in the bedroom. I started grabbing at our belongings and stuffing them into the bag. I already had a bag on standby which held most of Christopher's things, as the consultant had previously suggested I kept this. I grabbed a quick shower and got dressed, threw together a comfortable ensemble, and started chanting instructions to Kevin. "The bags are by the front door. The pushchair is in the hall. They need to go in the car."

Kevin was awake and dressed now, already ahead of me in the planning. He ran down the road quickly to his parents' house, knocked on the front door firmly, waking them up. He quickly explained the situation. Howard, his father jumped out of bed and got dressed immediately: he was our transport to the hospital. Kevin went to the car and started running it to help defrost it. He had his coat buttoned up against the cold and was wearing his woolly hat. He set the blow-heaters on full and commenced scraping the windows, his warm breath showing in the frosty air.

I glanced out of the window and a passing thought flashed through my mind. Life is about to change again. I shook my head and focused on gathering Christopher's medication and his comforters. I took one last look around Christopher's room before scooping him up from his cot into my arms. I kissed him on his forehead and held him tightly wrapped in his blankets. I grabbed Christopher's snuggle toy and made my way to the top of the stairs. Christopher stayed fast asleep in my embrace. I took each stair slowly, making my way down towards the front door which is directly at the foot of the staircase. By now, Howard and Kevin were sat outside awaiting their precious cargo and his Mum.

All the bags were already safely stowed in the boot of the car. I leaned into the rear of the car and placed Christopher securely into the car seat, double-checking that the clasp was fastened. I made my way round to the other side of the car and sat on the bench seat next to Christopher, while Kevin locked the front door.

As soon as Kevin was in the passenger seat, Howard took to the road. "Bloody hell Dad, I did not get my seat belt on yet!" Howard didn't even acknowledge Kevin's remark.

Through the car window, the moon, large and full on this clear night, proudly took centre stage. Millions of stars sparkled like the backing dancers of a world-famous popstar playing at Wembley Stadium. Our journey was short. We arrived at the hospital well within the timeframe that the Sister had requested.

Kevin started to unload our belongings and gather the bags from the boot of the car. My nerves were getting the better of me. I stepped out of the car, all extremities shaking not just from the cold air but from apprehension of the events about to unfold. Howard came around to my side of the car and lit a cigarette to calm himself, even if he wouldn't admit it. He was extremely fond of Christopher: their bond was incredibly close. He was loving, caring, and full of fun just like any grandad should be. He would tease Christopher whenever possible.

I shut the car door quickly, keeping in the warmth for Christopher while Howard took long nerve-soothing drags on his cigarette, blowing plumes of smoke high into the sky. He took my hand and gave it a reassuring squeeze. "We've got this," he said, releasing my hand.

Kevin returned to the car after dropping off our belongings to the ward. Howard extinguished his cigarette. Kevin reached for the car door handle and opened it. I swiftly bent in and unclipped Christopher from his car seat, taking him in my arms again. Looking into my beautiful brave boy's eyes, I saw that he had stirred from his sleep as the cold air nipped at his nose. I placed him in his carrycot and started making our way towards the hospital doors.

With every step, I took in another feature of his adorable face. His blue eyes sparkling brightly like the stars in the sky we'd seen on the journey towards the hospital. The expression painted upon my baby boy's face: one of expectation and relief. Every step was one closer to his reckoning. As we neared the entrance to the ward, I looked down at my him and whispered, "Everything is going to be all right now – the doctors will make you better. I promise."

I pressed the button near the ward door and the door opened. We were met by the nurses awaiting our arrival. One nurse quickly took Christopher out of his carrycot and told us that he was going to one of the main specialist's rooms at the end of the ward. She explained that the room was cleaned and sterile ready for Christopher's arrival. The nurse instructed us to wash our hands and to attire ourselves in aprons and gloves, explaining that we should always do this before entering the room. She also advised us to change them regularly in order to limit the spread of infections.

We all took the advice and started to wash our hands and acquaint ourselves with the correct gloves and aprons while a nursery nurse made a start on unravelling Christopher from his blankets and his layers of clothing. Once Christopher was settled in the cubicle the nurses kindly asked us to wait outside. While we were waiting outside, the nursing staff commenced their normal pre-procedure protocol of checking Christopher's weight, temperature, blood pressure, and performing numerous blood tests.

Once these observations were complete, the sister returned with the consultant, transplant surgeon and specialist anaesthetists. The transplant surgeon commenced detailing the risks and possible complications of the procedure along with the expectations of the procedure itself.

While we were lingering on the transplant surgeon's every word, the anaesthetist started routine checks, recording the results on Christopher's notes, before explaining her role during the upcoming procedure.

The consultant also explained his role along with his action plan, including how they were keeping the donor kidney healthy while waiting for Christopher's results. He also observed and poked at my brave boy himself. I couldn't help thinking that my Christopher was being prodded and poked like a piece of meat sat on the butcher's shop counter. I knew their examinations were necessary, but his small fragile body was mottled from the change in temperature from his snug cot to the hospital ward.

Lying there, waiting for life-saving surgery, he looked so young and delicate, without a care in the world, unaware of the obstacles ahead of him.

Kevin always handled these situations far better than me: he asked all the questions – the how's, the why's, the where's and the when's.

My mind always went blank at these crisis times, or wandered off to the worst-case scenarios. So, I concentrated on soothing our courageous baby boy. I stroked the crease at the top of his button nose, his eyes blinking in slow motion as I applied the smallest of pressures to comfort and reassure him. His little chest rose and fell rhythmically with each breath. His fine hair shone like a spun golden thread sewn into the richest fabric of royal garments.

Suddenly the atmosphere changed: the air became thick with anxiety. Silence fell all around us and the only sound I could hear was the whirring of my thoughts. The theatre trolley appeared, accompanied by nurses. One nurse carefully lifted Christopher onto the trolley. The cold of the thin black cushion made him wince as his barely dressed body lay effortlessly upon it.

The nurse collected his notes and placed them at the foot of the trolley, checked that the signatures on the bottom of all consent forms were mine and that I was still happy for the surgeon to proceed with the operation.

I nodded my head as that was all I could manage. My knees were knocking together. I was sure they sounded louder than the wheels turning on the trolley now wheeling along the colourful corridors decorated with cartoon characters, and tranquil scenes of rainbows unicorns and butterflies. My body was jolting with fear, my hand shook so much that the bottle of water I was carrying looked like a storm trapped within the plastic.

The porter raised the metal handrails on the trolley.

Kevin and I slowly walked behind, passing all the medical staff along the way. They all knew us all well and wished us good luck. Their eyes had a depth of empathy towards us as parents, understanding what it was to endure the process of kidney transplantation on such a young child – only eighteen months old. Some of the nurses were parents themselves, imagining how we must be feeling at this moment.

We walked along the long, cold corridor, with only the decoration adorning the walls to warm the space. Kevin steadied me, holding my arm as we walked.

The silence was complete until we arrived at the theatre doors. The theatre staff then re-checked all details including

Christopher's hospital number, his date of birth, and all other checks. Then came those words: "Would you both like to give your little one a kiss and tell him that you love him?" Obviously, we both did this.

Kevin suggested that I should stay with Christopher while they started to put him under general anaesthetic, a suggestion the nurse agreed with. I took hold of Christopher's small hand pressing my fingers into his grasp, gently kissing the top of his beautiful head. His perfect little body quickly became heavy, and with a few jolts of his body, the anaesthetic took hold. He became limp and restful.

I gave him another kiss before the nurse escorted me out of the theatre, doing her utmost to comfort me during the short walk. As we reached the door, I met Kevin and Howard. Kevin wrapped his arms around me tightly while I cried into his chest, creating a wet patch of tears and snot on yet another of his tops.

We made our way back to the ward where there was a comfortable room, purpose-built for trying to comfort parents. I wiped at the tears dripping from my chin. Howard sipped from his coffee cup.

We waited for what felt like forever for any news from the theatre. Nurses popped into the room, sporadically checking on our welfare, offering to provide refreshments and magazines.

Time went slowly, yet the sun rose, filling the room with natural light. So many thoughts raced through my mind, including the plans for Christmas dinner. We had been planning to go to Kevin's parents for lunch. However, that didn't seem likely now. It looked as if we might have to spend Christmas in hospital.

CHAPTER 3

A failed transplant

The door swings open and a nurse says our names. I stand up vigorously, kicking over Kevin's coffee. Kevin was looking at me with annoyance but at that exact moment I noticed the nurse had entered the room. However, what was more apparent was the tone of her voice. Even my body noticed the change in the atmosphere, every hair on my skin was poised for something dreadful. You know that reaction in your body: when the music changes in a scary movie or when the room suddenly turns deafeningly motionless.

My heart was thumping like a rabbit trapped in a cage, beating quicker than a train passing through Piccadilly. The Nurse then speaks once more but my ears are too scared to hear her and they block the sound from her lips. She then walks towards me with her delicate hand reaching out for mine. She repeats her words. Christopher is out of theatre now and is comfortable in his bed on the ward. If you take a few moments to gather yourselves you may go and sit with him. Although, I must warn you, he may wake up groggy and in some discomfort. It's important to try to keep him still and calm.

I was out of the room like a shot. I remember thinking that the worrying was all in my head. My thoughts running away with me, playing tricks with me. Christopher looked so sweet and calm, my brave boy was so peaceful and still.

There was another nurse, younger than the first. Fresh from a goodnight's sleep, you could tell, with a hue of fragrant perfume with a hint of musk. Eyes wide as the sun framed by mascara and eyeliner simply drawn on to open the eyes further. Her perfect complexion fit for the big screen. Her hair secured back with bobby pins and a net. Her smile flashing her pearly whites, and lips as smooth as velvet.

Her comforting words flowed from her lips with the ease of the breeze on a summer's day calming the searing heat.

She was perched in front of a raised surface at the foot of Christopher's bed. All Christopher's charts were sprawled across it. Every few moments she glanced at all the monitors on the machines.

She took a lingering look at me. I asked "What's wrong with my baby? Why are you having to stay in the room like this? Is this normal? What does that machine do? Why is my baby hooked up to that?" All these questions did not faze the young nurse, but I think she sensed my concern. After all, I normally have no questions, Kevin is the one that questions everything.

The young nurse moved from her seat for a moment and glided over to me. She then explained that for at least the next 48 hours Christopher would be receiving 1-to-1 observation. She further explained that once the transplant surgeon and consultant had finished in the theatre and written up their notes, they would be in to explain the procedure and what to expect next.

She then checked Christopher's temperature and pulse, then returned to her stool.

With that Kevin and Howard appeared in the open the door. Howard's head, just through the gap, asked: "Is it ok to come in, love?" to the nurse. I smiled thinking once a charmer always a charmer, our Howard! The young nurse replied: "Only if you're quiet and good...my grandma warned me about men like you". Howard's eyes sparkled as he threw me a look as if to say "bloody hell, I'm in trouble before I start!"

The men then made themselves comfortable on the chairs provided on the left-hand side of Christopher's bed. I could see them both studying the readings on the machines, which were making noises like a brass band at practice. Some bum notes, some in tune, yet, when put together making the melody of a well-rehearsed orchestra. The bleeping of the machines, the ticking of the clock, the vacuum of the ventilator and the whistle of the breathing mask.

All of which have their role to play in allowing my brave son to recover from the kind of ordeal that, hopefully, most 18 months old children will never have to endure.

Suddenly feelings of complete anguish and fear travelled through my body. I grab for the right hand of Christopher to soothe myself using his touch. His hand was warm and small with the smallest of wrinkles in his skin, from where it had lain on the creases in the sheets.

I start to stroke the back of his hand. Those feelings are overwhelmingly strong. The music of this nightmare movie is even now ringing in my ears.

I felt a kind of impending doom, like when Jaws circles the boat, thrashing his weight around in the sea before he breaks through the ocean wall, his jaws open wide. Then crash ... a boat broken into pieces and the blood of the victim dispersing in the sea. (I know you all have that theme tune ringing in your ears now, and if you don't: google it). Anyway, getting back to those feelings.

Just as my knees started to buckle, the young nurse stood to attention and the transplant specialist and consultant, along with the sister of the ward, saunter into the room.

This time there was a sense of concern in their glances towards each other. You could tell they had rehearsed who was going to be a good cop or bad cop. The one who would break bad news, then the other was going to talk options.

Sure enough, I was right. My brave boy had just undergone surgery that was supposed to change his life for the better. Never did I allow myself to imagine that it could turn out this way. My beautiful little soldier lay limp in the bed while the professionals talked about options and realities and whatever else they decided might make things better. How could they make things better?

My son. The very boy that I should protect, the one I should hold, see grow up, watch walk through the school gates, and wave to on his first school trip, not this. This was not what it should be like. My tears flow faster than the waterfalls of Dyserth after a torrential downpour. My heart yet again pounding. The strength in my muscles fading to weakness. Howard scoops me up and escorts me from the room to catch my breath.

We walk through the brightly coloured corridor, my eyes stinging from the tears, my breathing short and rapid.

Howard was so caring, even though he was a joker most of the time. I know that at this very moment his heart is breaking too.

Kevin stayed in the room where the transplant specialist explained every moment of the operation. They explained that the operation went like clockwork right up until the process of closing Christopher's tiny body. Before closing an incision in theatre, they use an ultrasound scanner to show blood flow to the kidneys. This is when the whole procedure started to unravel.

The surgeon then investigated the issue. It was confirmed by using a probe that the blood flow to the donated kidney was non-existent. The vein carrying the blood was completely blocked (this is better known as Deep Vein Thrombosis or DVT). This, unfortunately, caused the donor kidney to fail.

As a mother I cannot even begin to imagine the feelings that Kevin was facing while in that room all alone. Well, as alone as he would ever feel. I had Howard propping me up, holding me tight, bringing me comfort in my hour of need, but all Kevin had was a room of professionals assessing his every movement and reaction. Kevin told me afterwards that the young nurse did attempt to comfort and reassure him.

But knowing Kevin as I do, he was raging inside, hurt by his powerlessness to make a success of what should have been his son's life-changing operation.

The guilt that we have both felt during the process of the last 18 months never seems to disappear it was always lurking around the next corner, always hiding in the shadows. Everyone has an opinion on our boy's health. What is best for him. What is not best. But we are his parents: why is it we have so little to give our boy in the moments he needs it the most?

We have both hit ourselves with the "guilty stick" on numerous occasions. Sometimes these moments lead us to frustration, and at other times they lead us to strength. But we forget that it's not our feelings that count right now. The health of our brave little boy, who is now laying there oblivious to what's going on around him, is paramount.

I turn to Howard as I wipe the sodden tissue across my cheek, drying the stray tears rolling down my face. The cuffs of my jumper are soaked with tears, snot, and whatever else I used them to wipe away. "I'm ok now, we should get back to see what's next for our boy." I take a longer than normal cleansing breath and turn my body towards the entrance of the hospital. Howard extinguishes yet another cigarette.

Howard took my arm and linked it with his, saying: "Come on girl, we can do this as long as we all stick together. Christopher won't give in that easy, neither can we!"

Off we go back along the beautifully coloured long corridor. My life revolved around these corridors, though every step I take along them feels like the first, never knowing what's going to come to light after every step.

The consultant was just leaving Christopher's room as we entered. He said: "I have fully explained to dad the unfortunate circumstances. I will give you both a while to gather your thoughts and if you have any questions, I will do my utmost to find the solutions". Howard extended his arm shaking the hand of both specialists and consultants. His way of saying thanks.

We all sat in silence and again listened to the noises like a brass band at practice, some bum notes, some in tune, yet, when put together making the melody of a well-rehearsed orchestra.

The bleeping of the machines, the ticking of the clock, the vacuum of the ventilator and the whistle of the breathing mask all working together. Just like each one of us with a role to play in this nightmare called life.

After a short thinking period, I muttered quietly, "What happens next?" Kevin shrugged his shoulders and remarked maybe we should ask the consultant after he has managed to grab a bite to eat. "He said he needed a coffee and a sweet treat," said Kevin. "Maybe we all do", sighed Howard. "I will stay here in case Christopher wakes up", I answered. "Be a love though, bring me back a tea and chocolate bar".

Christopher was still motionless, still unaware of the sadness and anguish surrounding his bed. I sat watching every dimple, every breath in and every breath out. I watched as the creases in his eyelids fluttered and his lips parted so very slightly.

I noted the shape of his nose and the way his hair grew with a natural flick. I made a mental note of the smell of his forehead when I kissed him slowly. His fingernails sharp like needles on the smallest hand. The bruising appearing from where the surgical tape was holding the tubes in place.

Every fifteen minutes the nurse made observations of his temperature and pulse while she studied his complexion and asked if this mark on his cheek is normal or something new. I remember him hitting his cheek at home when getting excited with a toy in his hand after me telling him to be careful, for the tenth time. Her reply was sweet and comforting. "He is a remarkable little boy, a true fighter. You should be immensely proud." I was indeed so enormously proud.

The smell of fresh coffee and sticky buns meets my nose and soothes my spiralling senses. The comfort of Kevin and Howard reappearing with their hands full. I take my tea and iced bun and place them on the surface at the side of the room. Kevin throwing a sarcastic remark: "Try not kicking this one, I'm running out of change for the machine."

"Dad and I have been thinking of things to ask the consultant," said Kevin, as his bum takes to the seat, making an inappropriate noise. Embarrassed, he explains "that was the chair love" to the young nurse. "Yeah, and pigs will fly," said Howard. The consultant then enters the room asking if we'd had time to think yet. Kevin nodded. "What happens next?"

The consultant explains: "In the first instance we would like to monitor Christopher for the next 2 weeks to allow his body to fully recover from the surgery and secondly to allow us to monitor the function of his existing kidney. Then if his kidney is working sufficiently, we should be able to allow him to come home keeping him under close observation via our outpatient service. Does that sound ok for you?"

Kevin then asked "What about another transplant? Is that possible? Would it fail again?"

"Good question. Transplantation is a possibility. However, Christopher is unable to be placed back on the transplant list until he reaches 2 years old. He would require a donor kidney from a baby. As you already know, we can't give a time frame for a donor. Christopher could be waiting quite a while."

Our thoughts all-consuming, we say thanks to the consultant and allow the news to sink in. We simultaneously reach for our hot drinks and sweet treats.

The consultant leaves after entering something in Christopher's notes. Howard starts chatting to the young nurse as he only knows how to either flirt or question. He asked her things like how long she has worked here. Does she have a boyfriend? It's rather cute considering he would never have a chance. Not that he was trying. It was more like a distraction technique. A well-timed and desperately needed distraction! Kevin sat as still as a mouse when it senses danger. His eyes are fixed on his little boy.

The days passed slowly. With every passing hour Christopher was starting to get stronger, recovering well after the operation. The young nurse was no longer at the foot of his bed. Christopher was now showing his character more and more.

The more I study this boy the more I find him enchantingly entertaining to watch. The way he studies his toys. The way he watches every movement of the medical staff.

This boy is going to be intelligent and is going to make everyone proud, I feel it in my bones. Call it a mother's intuition.

The way his eyes burn brighter when he sees something new or interesting. The way he frowns with the pain but never recoils. My boy is braver than I could ever be, though now he is as vulnerable as a delicate rose swaying in the wind.

A long few months pass as we await news of appointments and transplants.

Christopher gets stronger by the day even though you can see he's struggling. His tiredness affects his activities. His restless sleeping and his loss of interest in the things he enjoys. The constant onslaught of medication, blood tests urine samples and doctors and nurses prodding and poking at my him. But he doesn't even say "ouch" or cry out. He just has an understanding beyond his years of what is necessary to keep him going. If only we could receive a call soon.

That makes me sound extremely selfish because I know that this means that another mother has lost their perfect baby. The pain felt by one family and the willingness to do something life-changing for the good of another family. I couldn't be thinking about it.

My heart breaks every time, but I love my boy so deeply and I would give all that I have to make him feel better.

Sometimes I sit and think about what I would say to a grieving mother, but I draw a blank. After all, nothing would be enough to relieve the pain of losing your child. I understand the concept but I'm unable to accept it as a possibility unless there are no other options. I lie in bed at night promising to be a better person if my boy gets another chance, and soon.

CHAPTER 4
Transplant: Take 2

Here we go again. May 1988. At least the weather was warmer and the days longer. Another day of washing and cleaning the house with Christopher playing in the garden for an hour or so. A butterfly flutters around him to hear his captivated giggles. How infectious is a child's laughter? The delightful sound of their fun ringing through the daisies and the tulip-edged garden.

The smell of the freshly laundered clothes swaying in the warm breeze. The humming of the busy world. The traffic charging from A to B, travelling from the city to the outskirts of town. The neighbour's lawnmower startled Christopher so much that he waddles straight over to me, clinging to my skirt hem. I stifle my laugh as I scoop him up in my arms, resting him on my hip and explaining to him what made the noise. He clings to the fence, fascinated by the neighbour cutting his grass in perfectly straight lines like those found in council parks or bowling greens.

"Soon be time for tea," I say to Christopher. I put him back down and settle his wobbles with my hand. We both walk into the house holding hands, unsuspecting of what is about to happen, blissfully ignorant of what the next 24 hours will bring. I settle Christopher in the lounge and make my way upstairs to run him a bath. He is a proper water baby who loves splashing around in the bath and being in there until the water gets cold or his skin wrinkles.

The day draws to a close and an early night is had by all. A warmer night than normal. I toss and turn restlessly in bed, finally settling just after 11 o'clock. The next thing I notice is the ringing of the phone. I jump quickly out of bed, grabbing my dressing gown, stumbling down the stairs to stop the blasted phone from disturbing Christopher.

I whispered "hello". In complete shock, I sat on the bottom step next to where the phone is secured. That voice that I'm so familiar with. I'm hearing it again on the other end of my phone. It was the sister from the kidney ward of Pendlebury Children's Hospital.

Her words are stern and authoritarian. "We have a match for Christopher. Collect your belongings and get here as soon as possible!" "See you soon", I reply before placing the phone on the receiver. A multitude of mixed emotions is swirling around my head.

Overwhelming emotions of happiness, that my brave boy was lucky enough to get another chance at life. Especially so soon after his first transplant failed. Flashbacks of that moment play over and over in my head day after day. The fear builds in my body, the knot growing tighter deep within my stomach. The anguish of it all. Am I even awake or is this just an extension of my nightmare? My skin grows clammy and my thoughts race. I rub my hand along the sleeve of my dressing gown.

I turn to walk back up the stairs and stumble. "Ouch!" I say under my breath as I stub my little toe. I must be awake, that hurt! In a flash, I realise the call I just received must have been real too. However, just to check I call the hospital back. The sister answers the call before it even seems to ring.

In a fleeting moment my voice disappears as my mind searches for the words. I explain who I am and the sister replies: "I was waiting for you to call back. I didn't think you were awake enough to understand what I was telling you before".

She then goes on to explain again that a match has been found for Christopher and we should make our way safely to the hospital, but being mindful the clock is yet again ticking. I know now that the call was not part of my imagination.

I return upstairs to collect Christopher's belongings, and call Kevin. Kevin no longer lives with Christopher and me. However, that's not for explaining now. This book is about the life and journey of my brave boy and after the last transplant failed it was all too real a possibility that the same thing could happen again.

My boy would be going through yet another risky procedure that could save his life, or could fail and become the very thing that might possibly kill him. I knew this was his last attempt and, even worse, his last hope.

Christopher was so happy only hours before, playing in the garden. I loved hearing his laughter fill the space in the back garden, watching him explore the wildlife of the butterflies and the bees as they playfully dance around the sweet nectar of the flowers. Dare I even say this, but my brave boy looked normal, without pain and without a care in the world. I know that was not an everyday thing and I know this was just a fleeting moment, however, it was a moment that I want to treasure and be able to see time and time again. My utmost love and protection for Christopher must also include allowing the doctors to help his failing body and have another last-ditch attempt at saving my baby boy.

The anguish in my tummy and the quickened beating of my heart builds as Kevin arrives at the house to collect us and take us to Pendlebury Children's Hospital once more. Christopher was very sleepy in his car seat and the journey seemed rather longer than last time. The thought fondly flashed through my mind like a gentle reminder. "Yes, but Howard was driving last time, Wendy, every journey is faster when Howard was behind the wheel!"

A small smile decorated my face, allowing me relief for a moment from my worries and fears. I longed to have the calming gentle nature of Howard by my side once more, but due to the recent break-up between me and Kevin, I knew that Howard would not be there this time to hold me together and bolster my nerves.

As we neared the hospital, I lifted my head and looked at the reflection of Kevin in the rear-view mirror. I shot him a look back. The air was quite thick and tense between us now, but I was trying hard to remember that he was here for his son and that should count for something.

Or was he trying to make out to the rest of the world what a doting father he was? I know differently, but he is here. I lift my head again and ask, "are you ok?" Kevin shrugs his shoulders. A man of few words. I could tell that he was not ok but too proud to say. I take Christopher's tiny hand and give it a gentle squeeze, enough for me to feel his warm fingers though not enough to wake him. I lean towards him and as my lips reach his forehead he stirs, opening one eye a little and then the other.

I sooth him with a gentle stroking motion across his forehead and down his nose. In that instant, my love poured out through the tears streaming suddenly from my eyes.

I reach for a tissue stashed away in my handbag, giving myself a gentle reminder: I should have sorted out my handbag the other day. I find a half-eaten packet of crisps, a lollypop without a wrapper, and a little toy car that I take everywhere for Christopher to play with while he is in his buggy.

Kevin searches for a parking space as close to the entrance as possible. I ask him to change spaces. He shoots me a look, asking, "what's wrong with here? I can't get any closer". I remind him that this was the exact space his father parked last time and look how that turned out.

My annoyance that he would not even think of this starts to show in my whole body. I take a deep breath and let out a long sigh while rolling my eyes, like a stroppy teenager.

I just wanted everything to be different, to give my brave boy the best chance. I know it's irrational but I will try everything. Kevin agrees to move the car and releases the handbrake, allowing the car to roll back into a neighbouring spot. "Is that any better for you?" he sarcastically asks while turning his body towards me to look me in the eye. I reply: "It will do". I reach for the door handle and clamber out of the car, slamming the door behind me. Kevin gets out, slamming his door too. He then makes his way to the boot to collect Christopher's belongings. I unbuckle Christopher from his seat and take him in my arms. My boy is still so small and featherweight.

While Kevin loads the buggy with Christopher's things, I decide to carry Christopher in my arms. I get to hold my boy tight to my chest and wrap my arms around him to create a protective shield while we walk with haste down the long winding corridor. Taking every step closer to the ward, my heart thuds and my pulse quickens, my eyes stinging from a mixture of lack of sleep and sobbing.

I cleanse myself with a deep breath and reach for the buzzer on the wall. Before I can announce our arrival, the door opens and we are escorted to the side room of the ward. The consultant and transplant specialist along with numerous nurses and the anaesthetist are all waiting to receive Christopher.

The nurse starts pulling at Christopher's clothing, taking off layers, and asking me questions about his last meal. What did Christopher last eat? When was that? When did he drink? How much? The questions were being fired at me from all directions of the room by all manner of persons. A nurse turns to Kevin and says you can answer these questions too if you like.

I quickly remark that it's good luck he is not around anymore. He likes playing happy families, but we are not. The atmosphere in the room instantly thickens, like when you are flying through the sky and suddenly enter the clouds.

The transplant specialist explains to Kevin and me that the protocol will remain the same as the previous attempt and this procedure should take around 2-3 hours.

He also explains that this could be Christopher's last attempt at a transplant. He asks if we have any questions and reassures us that he is rooting for Christopher, and for this time to be a success. I could see with every word spoken by the doctors, specialists, and nurses that Kevin's anxiety and fears were rising along with my own. My ears prick up at the familiar sound of the theatre trolley rolling through the corridor.

The consultant then asks for our consent to take Christopher to the theatre. I squiggle my name with my shaking hands and return his pen to him, my knees knocking and the tears flowing yet again. You would think that my tears would be dry by the time we had got here, due to the amount I have cried in the last two-and-a-bit years. Yet they still flow consistently, staining my face with their tracks.

Kevin stands on the side-lines, nervously taking in all the information being given in the room while watching over his boy's body. Christopher's body is being pulled and pushed, prodded, and poked with thermometers, blood pressure gauges, and needles.

Christopher looks so tiny and motionless on the bed while all these familiar faces take hold of a body part for this and a body part for that. The only sound from our boy is the yawn as he wakes from his slumber.

Once all the tests and recordings have been collected, we all wait with bated breath for the results being hurried through the labs. This makes for a tense time. I hate hanging around at the best of times. And waiting around for these results is somewhat, confusing for me. If they come back and say all ok to proceed then my boy is taken to yet another life-threatening procedure. My mixed emotions stir and twirl like a hurricane attacking the land, building in velocity as time goes by.

The footsteps of a determined nurse get louder as the deafening reality hits home. The results are in, I hear from afar. I hear her gather the porters and staff like a general gathering the troops ready to commence battle. *Surely my baby boy has battled on this field enough?*

The porters close in and the sister arrives at the foot of Christopher's bed. She says, "All good, and the theatre is waiting, let's go!" I gulp at the air around us as if it were my last breath. Again, I look deep into the eyes of my courageous boy and see calm.

This time though there seems to be a sense of him understanding what is happening around him. He searches the room with his eyes, still without sound or movement except for his eyes tracing the steps of his Mum. I am his warrior, his protector, his compass of knowing. We look at each other tenderly, with a deep sense of love and admiration for one another.

I hear a strangely familiar voice in the corridor of the ward asking for the room number for Christopher Simpson. A nurse replies with a warm greeting and escorts my mother into the room.

Christopher clocks the scent of his gran and rockets from his bed, arms raised, signalling to my mother that he needs her touch. The knowing touch of a loving, caring, (or rather doting!) Gran that she was. The bond between these two was picturesque and charming.

She is also my rock when I need strength. The last few months have been testing, to say the least, dealing with the heartbreak and split with Kevin. My mum has supported Christopher and me through it all, just like she will again today. The nurse asks who will be staying with Christopher while he is being put to sleep. Before I could even blink the words, "Mum, will you?" come out of my mouth.

My mum shrugged off her coat and laid it over the back of the chair. She made her way over to the sink in the room, washed her hands, turned to the nurse and said, "ready, where do you want me?" The nurse smiled: "Just follow behind the trolley with mum and dad and then when we get to the double doors, I will ask you to come through, once we have placed Christopher on the bed."

I shot mum a look. With no words exchanged she knew she was saving my ass yet again. This time though it was more for the love of Christopher, the apple of her eye, and I knew she would be the best person for the job. I could not go through that again. Off we stroll down this ever-expanding corridor towards the impending doom of the theatre and whatever was in store for us.

We reach the doors of Christopher's destiny and, with every inch of my will power I hold it together just enough to bend down and plant a lingering kiss on his warm soft forehead. I then tell him I love him and will see him soon. Kevin holds back not saying a word. He stroked the back of Christopher's hand while he was still on the ward, which was his way of wishing him well in his manly way. This was the emotionless robot that he had recently become.

We stood in absolute silence as the theatre doors open. Christopher and my mother disappear and the doors softly close again. This was like a tidal wave of emotions bursting from my eyes. I sobbed as the wait was agonising, the excruciating pain in my heart and head trawling through a mixture of thoughts as mum returns through the theatre doors.

The three of us walk back to the waiting room just like before. Kevin collects coffees and we all sit quietly with our thoughts. Mum now and again breaks the silence with a comment about the lady down the road or the shopping she needs to remember to add to the list. At one point she even vocalises her thoughts about taking a day trip to the beach when Christopher feels better. I loved her optimism, but I just wanted her to keep quiet, not because I couldn't see that far ahead but because it would cut deeper if I was to look forward only for things to turn out differently.

Time passes quicker than the last time we were here, or perhaps I caught up on some missed sleep. I do not recall noticing the sun rise, but it did as normal. Regardless of the struggling or the pain the sun always rises, the birds still sing their merry tune.

The nurse pops her head round the door with a friendly smile painted on her face with a muted pink shimmer. She informs us that Christopher is in recovery and will be with us shortly on the ward. I ask, "Is he ok? how did it go?" Her reply as courteous as ever: "the consultant will be through to see you once Christopher is settled."

I jump up and hug my mum. She is not as touchy-feely with her children as she is with Christopher.

Kevin lifts his head from the paper momentarily and says, "I will be through in a minute, you both go".

Mum and I sip the dregs of our drinks and hastily make our way towards the ward along the long, cold corridor still decorated with beautiful scenes of meadows and wildlife and the cartoon character that Christopher loves to watch.

As we wait in the room allocated to Christopher for the foreseeable future, he soon arrives back. His little body is tucked in by the tightly folded sheets. His eyes are closed, asleep, and peaceful. The nurse allows us both a moment to give him a welcoming kiss then asks us to step outside while she checks all Christopher's post-operative observations. She declares that she is also awaiting updates on the procedure.

The anxiousness rises in the room. Was this another failed attempt?

I stand opposite the door of Christopher's room, purposefully to see down the corridor towards the consultant's office, hoping to catch a glimpse of his demeanour. Will seeing him give me a clue to the outcome? My mum glares at me, shooting a remark: "I know what you are up to, my dear," she says scornfully, "I have seen that look before... you are trying to apprehend the consultant". I roll my eyes at being caught out. A mother always knows her child best. Even when they are grown up with their own children.

The nurse then signals her completion of Christopher's observations and we make our way back into his room. The consultant enters the room at the same time. We all take our respective seats. The nurse sits at her station at the foot of the bed, watching closely over Christopher's body and the attached monitor screens.

Again, we listened to the noises of our brass band at practice. Some bum notes, some in tune, yet, when you put them all together, making the melody of a well-rehearsed orchestra. The bleeping of the machines, the ticking of the clock, the vacuum of the ventilator and the whistle of the breathing mask all working together to fulfil their roles in keeping our brave boy alive and well.

The consultant explains that the new kidney had not woken up yet, reassuring us this was fine and to be expected. So why did it feel like another failure?

The consultant explains that the kidney is getting positive blood supply and that all signs were looking good so far. He explains a sleeping kidney sometimes just takes a while to start functioning fully. He tells us that, as before, Christopher is going to be under close observation 24/7 for the next 2 weeks. If we have any concerns, or if there are any early indications that the kidney is struggling, they will investigate and in the worst-case scenario, a biopsy will be done.

He seems optimistic and stresses that all the signs are good, so we should relax and allow Christopher's body to rest and recuperate. He finishes with: "It wouldn't hurt for the adults to rest too. Don't underestimate the impact on your well-being".

I think we all sighed a sigh of relief together, so much so that the nurse made a quirky comment, along the lines of "...and breathe...!". You could feel the electricity in the room, the positive vibes flowing from our pores. I was visualising the sunny beach days that Mum talked of earlier, and when I close my eyes, I can even feel the sand between my toes as I scrunch them up in my shoes. I so wished my boy could catch a break and be given a real shot at normality. Well, there would always be the medication, but it was a far cry from what we were facing otherwise.

Kevin rises suddenly and strides out of the room. Mum mutters something about him under her breath, but at this time I don't care about all the pain he has caused. At this very moment I want to squeeze my boy tight in my arms and hold him close.

We stayed by Christopher's bedside all day. Kissing him gently time and time again. My mother was the first in his eyeline. Of course she was, why did that not surprise me! Christopher stirred and started to regain consciousness and wiggle.

This child never did stay still for long. His monitor made an unusual sound. The nurse shot from her seat and reset the machine after checking Christopher's connections. He had knocked off his connector while wiggling. Nothing to be alarmed at.

The nurse was regularly checking his pulse, temperature, blood pressure, and his catheter for signs of the kidney starting to function. She made notes and took regular break intervals while another nurse would sit with us.

It was nearing 7 pm and the nurse had mentioned the shift change.

Christopher was again going to have a personal nurse assigned to sit at the foot of his bed throughout the night, taking the same measurements and observations. The nurse suggested I go home and get some rest.

They would call me if there were any changes, or if Christopher became unsettled.

She explained they would expect Christopher to keep sleeping, while his pain relief need was so high, and with his body needing to concentrate on recovery. I spoke to Mum and asked her to contact Dad who would come and collect us from the hospital. She stood and made way for the door as the consultant came in to wish Christopher and us good luck and goodnight. He said that he would be back in the morning, bright-eyed and bushy-tailed.

My mother, being her usual self, shot him a risqué remark, making me blush at the very thought. The consultant shot one almost immediately back to her and I just shook my head to erase it from my memory. We stayed till after 8 pm before I kissed my brave baby boy farewell.

On the way home I felt strange. I was going back to an empty home. No Kevin to distract my mind, and Christopher was in hospital. I had some washing to iron and put away and I could run the hoover over the living-room floor, but I knew I would be better off if I had company.

I asked Mum if I could go back home to their place for the evening. My mum was as sarcastic as ever: "I think I have had enough of seeing your face for one day," she said.

We picked up a chippy tea on the way home, just as dad pulled up outside my house. They asked me to put the kettle on and make them a brew. "We will dirty your plates and eat this here with you," they laughed. "Then you get something else to do to distract you for a while whilst you're washing the dishes," said Dad.

After tidying up and having a soak in the bath, I call the hospital, checking on Christopher's progress and get into bed around 10.30 pm. I slept like a log, which was unusual for me. I didn't have to listen out for Christopher in his bed. I woke early with the birds singing in the trees and the sun burning brightly in the bluest of skies, not a cloud in sight. The grass was a luscious green and felt like soft velvet under my bare feet as I peg out the sheets from my freshly laundered bedding. I pack some fresh pyjamas and Christopher's favourite comfort blanket along with a book we enjoy reading together.

I checked with the hospital how Christopher was doing this morning and if he had enjoyed a settled night, which he had. I told the nurse to expect me around 10 am and to tell Christopher I love him and would see him soon.

I finish up a few chores and call Dad to collect me to take me back to the hospital. Dad was very quickly at the house to pick me up.

He sounds the horn to signal his arrival. I collect the bags that I packed to take to Christopher and make my way to the car.

Getting into the car, my dad and I greet each other with a kiss on the cheek. My dad and I briefly chat, killing time on the way to the hospital. He pulls up at the door, giving me a message to pass on his love for Christopher. He then reminds me that he and Mum will visit later and take me home again. He then asked if I wanted a dinner cooked for me to take home for my tea. As if I'm going to refuse a meal from home! There's nothing like home-cooked meals from Mum. I shot him a smile and collected my bags from the back seat of the car, shut the door and waved goodbye.

I make my way confidently towards the ward, stopping at the little kiosk shop to buy a woman's magazine and a packet of Polo mints.

I then make my way through the cold corridor of the busy hospital. The hospital has a familiar hum of business and anticipation. The staff hurry from one place to another.

Children hold the hands of their parents as they skip through the corridors. Doctors glance down at pagers and talk to colleagues. The porters are all pushing beds or retrieving trolleys and wheelchairs.

I sense the distant sound of a disappointed parent, and the laughter and excitement of those with positive outcomes, the giggling of nervous children as they embark on unknown journeys.

The brightly coloured walls and the huge expanses of finger-print covered windows. The smells of stale coffee and cigarettes. The sweetness of fresh fruit on the newspaper trolley rolling past with Sue, the busybody of the town, her tabard unbuttoned and her shoes squeaking, her friendly smile warm and inviting. Her hair was always fresh from her heated rollers.

A lady I had met at one of Christopher's appointments a few weeks ago was walking towards me. We both clock each other simultaneously, cheerfully saying "Hi!" and enquiring about each other's visit today. Both our boys had been admitted on different wards. We wished each other well and arranged to meet for a tea break after lunch in the hospital café.

I carry on my journey along the corridor, finally reaching the doors to where Christopher is residing. I press the buzzer and the sister greets me at the door. She ushers me into the room where Christopher is sitting up in his bed, his eyes sparkling and his smile wide. "Mummy!" he says. My heart skips with hope and happiness.

Christopher's complexion was bright and glowing. He was excited and full of energy. My eyes filled with the most joyful and happiest of tears. Pride filled my whole body and reverberated through my bones. I felt on top of the world and tremendously proud of my brave baby boy. I could feel the weight disappear from my shoulders and the fog clear from my brain. The nurse shot me a smile a thousand miles wide, brightly outlined with amethyst lips. She beamed as she read me the notes of Christopher's recovery and his reactions to his new kidney.

Then she points to the bag attached to the catheter, with its fresh output. My heart leaps as the consultant arrives to explain his findings. He says we should proceed with caution and not celebrate too soon.

However, all the signs are pointing in the right direction and he says that Christopher is responding better than he thought he would at this early stage in the recovery.

This professionally skilled man then puts his hand on my right shoulder and says: "Mum, go give your brave boy some cuddles, I think you could both use them right now!"

I was over to Christopher's bedside in one fell swoop.

CHAPTER 5

Starting Nursery

Today is one of those days. Up until now, I could only have dreamt of such a day, considering all the circumstances that have been set before us. Suddenly, reality sends shimmers of hope our way. Most people dream of fame, others dream of a huge lottery win, swimming with dolphins or marrying the love of their lives. Yet my minuscule dream, enthralled with sadness and anguish, is beginning to feel less like a nightmare unravelling in the late summer breeze, and more like a vision of Christopher's life beginning to take a positive direction.

This is something we have all been determined to witness: his first day at nursery.

My whole experience of Motherhood has been a multitude of twists and turns of ever-changing directions. The harsh challenges of Christopher's health battles. The desire to see him live through the normal aspects of childhood. To see my brave baby boy set out on the beginnings of his educational journey.

The excitement fizzing through my veins can only be compared to the time when I peed on the stick of Cupid's extended arm (known to others as a pregnancy test). I say it could be compared to that time because I had similar feelings of excitement and nerves, trepidation, and worry, though,

I vaguely remember the awful sickly feeling when the second line appeared on that test.

This was not due to the fear of having a baby, but rather the fear of whether I could be good enough to be a Mother, with all the expectations of my distant teenage dreams.

All was rosy when I thought Motherhood would be like pushing an Angelique dolly through fields of yellow buttercups and the brightest white daisies, all the time listening to the mellow tunes of Jeffery Osborne's "On the Wings of Love" and other popular, soulful, idealistic songs.

I sometimes think of a couple at the beginnings of life, creating another human in the hour of lust and time of passion, yet momentarily forgetful of the consequences, taking the risk of a lack of contraception.

However, I would not change the outcome of that momentous occasion as my beautiful boy was created. He fills my heart with pride minute after minute. He is the very reason I breathe and fight the battles fate bestows on us.

Like the battles fought on fields full of inspirational, selfless, dedicated soldiers, our battles have been fought on hospital wards and with medication.

This boy, so plucky and strong, taking his first solo steps into his future independent of his mother. He knows I'm there giving him encouragement and reaffirming promises. I will walk every step beside him, standing strong and dedicated to his every breath.

Christopher, buzzing like the bees gathering the last of the summer nectar. Busy, energetically full of anticipation and zest for life. He keeps telling me that he "loves me" as he learns to read my thoughts and feelings.

On this first nursery day, I straighten the clothes that have become crumpled within seconds of covering his fragile body. His trainers are Velcro tight, securing his narrow feet to help preserve his balance as he rushes through the rooms at home, imitating the noises of car engines and the planes whooshing through the skies.

I check the list, posted to us before Christopher's first session.

Kevin and I had also previously met with all key staff members to explain Christopher's extenuating circumstances regarding his health. I shared my worries and fears about the impending separation we were both going to endure.

The nursery staff were mesmerised by the true grit and determination of such a young boy and his dedicated family. I was satisfied by their alterations to the nursery setting and the accommodations they had made to welcome Christopher into the weird and wonderful world of pre-school.

Christopher will only be attending pre-school for half days but that is far more than anyone expected only a few months ago.

We made our way towards the nursery just a short walk along the streets. Christopher pulling at my wrists, signalling me to walk faster and faster. His whole being filling my heart with happiness and admiration. How can this boy, so precious and fragile, live with so very few expectations and have a heart filled with a zest for living when all his young life he has had to fight for every victory?

We get closer to the Nursery and Christopher's excitement spills from his pores. This contagious ball of energy smiles as bright as the sun, yet his charming nature and inquisitive soul are thirsty to explore the mythical surroundings called 'nursery'. The presence of strangers, and other children, do not fluster this brave soldier.

We enter the nursery gate, Christopher like an excitable puppy being released from the shackles of the leash taking his first steps to freedom with the bigger dogs in the park, bounding from my side as soon as the nursery door opens.

Christopher strides straight through the nursery doors, passing the coat hooks and washroom. He made his way to the sand and water table just like I knew he would.

The nursery staff greet me with their friendly nurturing manner. Smiles and enthusiasm in abundance.

I glanced over to Christopher. He was already acquainting himself with children and adults, his little mouth moving quicker than his brain could keep up with. I smile at the odd little gasp for air as he struggles to get all his words out before someone else can get a word in.

This remarkable boy, so confident and engaging, everyone's favourite little fellow. Laughing and smiling, his body radiates energy, demanding the attention of adults and children alike. Not a care in the world for me, sat there in the room alone in my thoughts, the swirling of emotions speeding through my head, the flashbacks of darker times and the flashes of brighter times to come for us all.

Safe to say Christopher loved every moment of nursery and couldn't wait to skip down the road at close of play to tell Gran all about his new teachers and his new friends and the water play and the painting.

My fearless boy was adjusting well to the next stage of his life. Hopefully this pleasurable time can last a while longer, giving us the welcome break we all so deserve. But not as much as my lovely son deserves to be happy.

The days pass us by, and the outpatient appointments keep us in check. Christopher is making steady progress. His medication is stable, along with our family life.

CHAPTER 6

Oh no! Mum is having a Baby

Life as we have known it for the last few years, is all about to change.

This change is far different from the kind we have been used to. Our family of two soon became a family of three. I found the love of my life, Joe.

He came from nowhere. Like a bolt of lightning. Bright and courteous, caring, and thoughtful. He filled a void in my life that I never really noticed was there until he swooped me off my feet. An Army soldier who has shown the deepest empathy towards the challenging and lonesome times that I had endured while caring for Christopher. The kind of challenges that were downright unfair most of the time. I mustn't grumble though, I have the most amazing little boy thanks to Kevin, but Joe was an entirely different kind of man. He was a gentleman, with all the characteristics of a trained serviceman.

Joe made all my days full of joy, showing me unconditional love, and understanding my flaws but still loving me regardless of them. His compassion and care for Christopher would prove harder for me at times. I would feel guilt towards Kevin. He should be the one hearing Christopher's laughter and teaching him how to ride a tricycle. He should be the one to wipe the sweat from Christopher's brow when the nightmares swept in. However, Joe did all these things in his unquestioning manner, without judgement, shame, or ridicule. This man has a big heart, full of kindness, love, and admiration for the woman that he has asked to marry.

Excitement takes over my body and makes an involuntary squeal as Joe mutters the words: "Wendy, please do me the honour of becoming my wife". I made the man sweat a little.

I took a moment to breathe in the glory of all our happy moments and said, "Yes! I would love to be your wife Joe, but just so you know, the number one man in my life will always be Christopher". Joe replied quicker than I could swallow.

"That's why you are so beautiful inside and out. I wouldn't want to change your bond with Christopher. I want to marry you as well as become a more permanent fixture in Christopher's life. Create a stable loving home for you both and maybe one day we could embark on extending the family, but no rush, hey!"

The next few months pass quickly, and the wedding goes without a hitch. Christopher even takes centre stage by walking me down the aisle.

Christopher's health was providing us with a much-needed glimpse of normality. The doctors are content with his progress and even lengthen the period between each follow-up appointment. My Mum is still the apple of Christopher's eye, along with his teachers and his friends from the nursery who accept his quirky ways and his elaborate stories. The staff watch him, fascinated by his strength and endurance, though his fragile frame betrays his determination at times.

Christopher gets tired quicker than the normal four-year-old, and the exhaustion of chasing the bubbles blown in the nursery garden after following the trail of traffic with the balance-bikes and scooters, is taking its toll on Christopher. It takes its toll on me to watch on in amazement as he carves his way through the hustle and bustle of nursery activities.

I seem to be getting so tired lately, and have started to notice a sickly feeling coming from the pit of my stomach. These feelings tell me something untoward is on the horizon.

My maternal intuition indicates a change in circumstances. My internal barometer is off the scale. Worry turns to fear. I check Christopher's body rigorously, looking for signs of illness. A rash, an indent, a blemish, a smell, anything to alert me of the impending downward spiral that my intuition was sensing.

I couldn't help but feel sad to think that all the positivity in our lives at this very moment was going to come crashing down around our heels. I had many sleepless nights while I agonised over what could be coming our way.

Then I started to feel sick most mornings, but I had convinced myself that I was literally worrying myself sick. My sense of smell became so sensitive that I could tell if Joe had walked past the pub, let alone stepped in for a cheeky half on the way home from the shops or his mates.

I rang my Mum, sharing my feelings and how scared I was of what was coming next. Especially if it indicated that Christopher getting ill was about to happen all over again. My Mum suggested two things: first calling Christopher's consultant to suggest that Christopher be seen as soon as possible to undergo checks; the second suggestion was to take a pregnancy test.

I laughed at that second suggestion! Mind you, mothers are rarely wrong. I mentioned what Mum had said on the phone to Joe when he got home. He beamed from ear to ear. "Well", he said, "there is only one way we will find out - you will need to pop along to the chemist tomorrow after dropping Christopher at school."

I sat quietly most of the evening while Joe was watching TV with his feet up, stretched out along the sofa. Meanwhile I sat in the armchair across the room, my thoughts racing. I was not sure how I would feel with either outcome of my worries. The thought of being pregnant leaves me feeling excited and giddy, though it also terrifies me to my very core. Bringing another baby into the world! All the challenges that we have gone through with Christopher, did I have the strength to go through that again. I think not.

The guilt of another baby suffering relentlessly sends shivers down my spine. On the other hand, having a child that would not have to endure the painful procedures that Christopher has had to endure would be good. But that too would leave me feeling guilty, for Christopher mainly.

I blink, a lonesome tear resting on my cheek.

I stand and make towards the kitchen to put a freshly bleached cloth over the work surfaces, affording me some alone time. Joe knew better than to ask me for a drink or pass him a packet of biscuits when I was bleaching my sideboards. It is the only time I know I can be alone with my thoughts. My mind was playing tricks on me, bringing me back to horrific thoughts of the possibility of Christopher becoming critically ill again.

I check on Christopher, just as I do every night, on my way to bed. I plant a lingering kiss on his forehead, as I have done since the day he came home. He was soundly asleep, cuddled in with his teddy and blankets, one leg hanging off the bed. As I get into bed, the call of nature demands another toilet visit, Joe rolling his eyes at me as he settles into the sheets.

I toss and turn as Joe and I find it particularly difficult to drift off to sleep this evening. Joe can sleep in seconds, usually, I think it's part of his Army training. Joe asks me numerous times what is keeping me awake. My reply never alters: "I just can't get comfortable and it's hot in here tonight". Joe then tuts loudly and says "hurry up, get comfortable, then I can sleep too. I have work in the morning, my sleep is most definitely needed".

It must have been shortly after this that I fell off to sleep. The next morning seemed to have risen before I could even dream.

Mind you, the morning still brought tears. Tears of excitement, fear, and happiness. Although my relationship with Joe has been fantastically magical, the result of yet again peeing on this stick leads to an intense mixture of feelings.

I wait for my Mum to visit so that she can give me the moral support I desperately need, regardless of the outcome. I can say without a doubt this was far more nerve-wracking than finding out I was pregnant with Christopher.

I think it was just after one o'clock in the afternoon when the doorbell chimed. Mum stood in the doorway.

"Well? Is it baby steps? Please tell me it's not our Christopher?"

My knees were knocking and a nauseous feeling was ripping through my body. "I don't know yet, I was waiting for you." Mum came in and turned on the cold tap, reaching for the kettle. I just looked at her in the kitchen from the doorway of the lounge and asked what she was doing. "Making a brew, it will help either way". I fuss around for my handbag with the prescription bag in, hiding the contents from prying eyes in the nosey neighbourhood where we live. Everybody knows everybody and all their troubles.

I go to the bathroom, taking the test along with me. I follow the instructions folded neatly in the box accompanying the test and then wait. I couldn't look. Mum shouts through the door: "Have you fallen in the lavvy or are you on the floor and need reviving?" Her humour is mostly a welcome distraction, but not this time. I looked at the windows on the pregnancy test: it appeared to have 2 horizontal lines. I couldn't remember what that meant, so I unfolded the instructions again. I think I held my breath for a second or two. Mum was right outside the door when I opened it.

She knew the result before I could bat an eyelid or mutter a word. Her arms wrapped around me and the sound of excitement burst from her lips.

She cradled my weak body for what seemed like an hour. It must have been that long as the tea she brewed earlier was now stone cold.

Safe to say Mum was over the moon, though she could see my struggle with the outcome.

My head filled with fear and concern. All the "what ifs" in the world flooded the space between my ears. My body, growing another human! Hopefully, another chance to get it right. Although I know it was not my fault that Christopher had suffered immensely with his health. The doctors can't explain the reasons for Christopher's struggles.

What I do know is that as soon as I contact the GP to record my pregnancy, I'm going to be hooked up to monitors while every medical professional will want a piece of my body for testing. I know it's going to be in the best interests of baby and me, but is it so wrong to want to have a day or two to allow my headspace to absorb this shocking news? I never thought I would have another child. I always worried about what happens if both of my babies are unwell. Which one would I deal with first? How would I cope, if Christopher got ill and needed me but I had another child to care for? As you can tell, my head sometimes consumes my mind with negative thoughts and obstacles. Yet at the same time, my heart is pumping love and excitement through my veins at a rate of knots.

Joe was going away for work the day after tomorrow, so I needed to tell him as soon as he came home. Joe always said we would have children together one day. I know he is going to be so proud and excited. So why do I have this dreaded feeling about telling him? Mum tells me: "For goodness sake, my girl, give your mind a break from all these worries and come and sit down and sip this sweet tea that I have made for you. It's good for shock and for worried new mothers. I heard it on the radio the other day in the hairdresser's." She then remarks, "talking about hairdressers you should book yourself in for a wash and blow-dry, make that man of yours treat you. He has a lot to answer for now you are carrying his baby and off he goes again for weeks on end!"

I decide to wait and see what the doctors advise me. I couldn't forgive myself if pampering caused this baby to be ill too. We both sipped our tea in utter silence, although you could hear the twin-tub working away in the kitchen and next door having some new fences fitted. So when I say silence I mean not talking. There's no such thing as silence in this street.

Mum finished her brew and checked the beautiful, gold-plated wristwatch that she had won at the bingo last week. She says, "you better wipe those tears, lovey, it's time to walk proudly along this street with your head held high. Our Christopher will be waiting for us to collect him from nursery. Go splash your face with water. We will pop into the shop and get our brave boy a treat, he will love that! We could meet Dad and

Joe after work tomorrow at the park if you're feeling up to it. Take some bread for the ducks, our Christopher loves feeding the ducks and getting his Grandad to push him high on the swings." I nod my head in agreement. I knew Christopher would love to go feed the ducks.

That evening when Joe returned from his training drills, I cooked his favourite meal, stewed steak, new potatoes, peas, and carrots. I also made sure there were at least two cans of his best bitter chilling in the fridge. Sometimes I think my man can smell his way home when I'm cooking. He always enters the house just as the potatoes boil. This leaves him just enough time to have a quick shower and change his clothes. If I'm lucky, he will scoop Christopher from the lounge and take him upstairs too. I always get lost in the moment when I can hear my boys chatting away to each other. Christopher idolises Joe, though I think the feeling is mutual with those two. I can hear Joe laughing, while Christopher seems determined to prove he can do whatever it is. "I can do it, I'm a grown-up now. Mrs Walker at nursery told me I'm not a baby anymore."

Life seems so steady, dare I say easy-going now. Christopher's health is as good as it can be. Joe and I are happily in love and enjoy life together. A lump rose to my throat, as the impending news I'm about to break to Joe stings my eyes and throat. The news could complete our family, or it could cause ripples of chaos.

I walked towards the stairs to shout up to the boys and I'm met by Christopher's face covered in shaving soap, and him smiling from ear to ear, quickly followed by Joe with shaving soap still on half of his chin. Joe shoots me a look with a twinkle in his eye.

"Christopher is a big boy now, Mummy, he wants to shave and splash some after-shave on to smell good for the ladies," says

Joe with the proudest smile decorating his face, though I could see the love pouring from his heart towards Christopher. I smiled with my whole heart. I shout up to them, "you two boys best hurry up, make yourselves look and smell good. Dinner will be on the table in five minutes. If you're late the lady of the house will be eating alone, and she will not care how good you smell, you will both have a clip around the earholes for making this fine woman wait. Come on, I'm starving!"

I turn on my heels as I hear the saucepan lid rattle in the steam-filled kitchen. I enter the kitchen in time for the boiling water to be spilling over the saucepan. I remove the lid and take the vegetables from the heat, straining them with the lid slightly off centre.

Carried away with my thoughts, enduring the heat from the steam-filled kitchen, I didn't hear the boys make their way downstairs.

I felt the warm and tender touch of Joe as he wrapped his arms tightly around my waist from behind, lowering his head to my neck, planting a kiss so gentle. My senses overloaded with the smells of the kitchen, layered with the rather giddy feelings of love and comfort when Joe wrapped his arms around me. Then there's the sight of my most prized possession, Our Christopher, my brave son. He looked so dapper with his hair slicked to the side, just like Joe, and his shirt tucked half into his trousers, again just like Joe. They were more like twins than stepfather and son. Christopher's eyes were the brightest blue, sparkling and accompanied by little giggles escaping his mouth as he shot Joe and me a look of pure admiration.

"Look at you two, who are the lucky ladies you are both trying to impress?" The boys just laugh out loud. Joe asked if I had got any cans for him. I point to the fridge as I move around our small galley kitchen.

I use a sequence of steps that to the onlooker could resemble a cha-cha or quickstep. I plate up the meals and leave Christopher's on the windowsill under the open window to cool off somewhat, while I carry Joe's meal and place it on the table along with my freshly poured chilled water from the tap. I then return to the kitchen for mine and Christopher's meal. The meal is, as usual, a time for us all to talk about our day. Christopher tells us about his day at nursery, and yet again how he played on his favourite scooter and then had a story about a family going on a bear hunt.

He loves nursery. As we finish our dinner, I tell Christopher to go look in the fridge. I watch him all the way. I see that he clocks that I have whisked up some Angel Delight for us in three small bowls.

Today does feel special. I still have news for them both. I keep taking lingering looks at both my boys, knowing our worlds are about to become crazily different, hopefully in a good way. The anticipation builds in the room. The atmosphere feels like a thunderstorm rolling in. The electricity building, I leave the table for the third time during our meal. I have a need to pee frequently. As I'm sitting in the bathroom, I decide I'm going to tell the boys when I return. I wash my hands and take a deep breath, place my hand on the door handle just as it turns in my hand. Joe appears: "Are you ok?" he enquires.

My eyes instantly burn with the tears pooling within them. I lift my head, looking him square in the eye and said, "I think I'm ok, I have something I need to tell you". He kisses me on the tip of my nose. "Baby", he says, "tell me what it is". I blurt out, "Joe I'm pregnant".

He grabs me swiftly, taking me off my feet, spinning me around and then holding me close to him with my feet still off the ground. "Really, baby?" he asks. I just nod as a tear spills down my cheek. "That's fantastic!" he says. He then sets me on my feet. "When did you find out?" "Today!" I reply. With that Christopher came running through asking if I was ok: "Mummy, why are you crying, are you sad?" I say, "Mummy will tell you in a minute, could you go wash your hands and come through to the lounge to Joe and me?" He is off in a zoom to wash his fingers.

Joe is holding my hand tightly. He keeps kissing me: "Really, baby, we are having a baby!"

He is made up. We sit on the sofa and Christopher comes speeding in, his small fingers still dripping with soapy water. He discreetly wipes them on his trouser legs. Joe lifts him onto his knee and sits there holding him so that he is facing me. "Mummy and I want to tell you something! Mummy has a baby in her tummy, you are going to be a big brother!"

Christopher looks at my face, studying my expression, he is such an intuitive little boy. "So why are you crying, Mummy? Do you not like the baby in your tummy? We can call the doctors at the hospital and ask them to take it out for you and make you better like me, Mummy". I smile and grab at him for a cuddle. I tell him, "Mummy is crying because I'm happy. I'm a little scared, a little excited, but mostly I'm happy!"

Christopher looked at Joe and then again at me: "Why do big people cry all the time? When you get bigger you shouldn't cry anymore. Only babies cry. Oh no, babies cry!!" He placed his hand on his forehead while he shook his head.

The next few months were filled with outpatient appointments with Christopher and then scans, blood tests and more scans for me and the baby. I felt like a pincushion with all the blood taken from me.

I suppose I had a sense of how my brave baby son must've felt while being in and out of hospital all those times. At least I understand why I need all these tests. It must've been so scary for my boy.

I was classed as a high-risk pregnancy, due to the complications that followed Christopher's premature birth and ongoing health challenges. Most of my appointments and scans were always followed by a consultant visit.

I recall that when I got to 22 weeks, whilst having another routine scan the consultant asked me if I wanted to know the sex of my baby. In total honesty, in my head I did want to know, though my heart was battling against me, telling me not to get too attached to this child in case something happened like last time, or even worse. Also, Joe and I had discussed finding out the sex of the baby before him going away again for work.

We had decided together that as it was his first baby we didn't want to know. If I'm honest I felt in real turmoil myself. At times I wanted to know, at other times not. Finally, I decided not to find out. At least we can both share the moment when the midwife who delivers the baby announces the news.

The pregnancy continued without any major issues, just the odd water infection and tiredness, but nothing to worry about. As the six-month mark came and went, along with the seventh month and the eighth, my nerves settled more and more, though with every twitch I would have a mini-panic. I would worry myself to sleep most nights.

Christopher was caring and gentle around me, getting more and more excited as time went by. He would tell anyone he ever met that I was having a baby. Not that I could hide this enormous bump growing at my front. He would say, "how much longer until the baby comes, Mummy?" I would reply: "Not too long!"

The final month was hard going, with tiredness and the aches and pains setting in. I was finding it increasingly difficult to get comfortable or rest. Walking Christopher to Infant School was a real struggle. Joe was due home in a week. I knew things would be easier. The last 3 weeks passed quickly.

The appointments were now every 3 days. Every possible check and test were done. To be honest, this baby was now outstaying its welcome! I remember sitting in the hospital waiting room thinking, "enough is enough, just pop out now so I can walk without a waddle and see my legs again, let alone paint my toes or climb the stairs without having to take a break halfway up!"

I grow more uncomfortable and impatient with every passing hour, though I feel different this evening. A mysterious feeling seemed to fill the air. I felt as if I should be resting though I was unsettled. I wanted to soak in the bath, then after the rigmarole of getting in, I felt like I was melting, claustrophobic, and wanted to get out.

I shouted for Joe to come and help steady me as I clambered from the tub. As he was walking across the landing, I had such an intense pain shoot from one side of my swollen tummy to the other. Beads of sweat were forming on my brow.

My tummy so tight, I take a deep breath, my eyes wide as I instantly remember these pains. "Joe!" I shout again. "Quick, the baby is coming!"

He bursts through the door, his face terrified, and I could tell by the look deep beyond his eyes he had no idea what to expect or do next. You would think that with all his army training he would be good under pressure. Ha-ha, not this time! He helped me from the bathroom and into the lounge. When the pains passed again, I started calling out the lists of things he needed to do, one of which was to call my Mum so that she and Dad could come over and look after Christopher. It was a mild evening for February, but still cold enough to bring flooding back the memories from when I was rushing to the hospital for the premature birth of Christopher.

As soon as Mum and Dad arrived, I was up from the sofa and out of the house. Joe and me, making our way to Fairfield General in Bury. Joe was driving carefully along the roads, nothing like when Howard drove me to Bolton General to have Christopher. I know situations were different now, but part of me was wishing that Joe would drive more like Howard, this baby is coming, and I don't want to be having it in the passenger seat of the bloody car! "Argh!" I squeal, with yet another contraction. "This baby is determined to make me swear", I shout to Joe as I try wriggling in the seat and using the breathing exercises taught to me in the anti-natal classes. Sweat is flowing down my back and face as if I had forgotten to dry myself from the bath. My cheeks were glowing rouge, my breath shortening as panic set in. My body was doing its magic, while my mind was busy playing tricks.

Finally, we arrive at the hospital. It was a busy evening. The maternity staff were awaiting my arrival. Joe grabs hold of my suitcase, which holds all the essentials needed for the next few days, nappies, changes of clothes for us both and not forgetting the breast pads.

Joe then parks the car and takes me hand. He sees the tears sparkling in the moonlight and tells me to stop crying, there's nothing to cry for, he is with me every step of the way. He then leans in for a kiss, so I snap at him telling him to get lost: "Joe, I need to just get in there!" pointing to the hospital. He asks if I need a wheelchair. I reply, "I will walk thanks". Taking the quickest paces my body would allow, I waddle towards the entrance of the hospital.

The corridor was awash with magnolia and light blue. There was a broad handrail to steady my nervous knees and lean against with each contraction. It was just a short walk until we arrived at the reception. You know when you have visited too often, when the staff don't even check your name or credentials, they just buzz the door and wave you through!

A midwife meets us at the door and escorts us past the waiting room full of labouring ladies and their eagerly anticipating partners. I am shown straight to a delivery suite with my consultant on standby and specialist midwife. Joe's face is a pale shade of grey. The midwife cracks a joke, asking "who is having this baby? Looks like Daddy is not feeling great!" I glance over to Joe and tell him to sit down before he passes out.

To spare you all the gory details, the birth went as smoothly as possible. Mother and baby were fighting fit. A beautiful baby girl named Claire Louise was born 21st February 1990, healthy without any complications.

Daddy, on the other hand, looked exhausted and drained but overcome with the most heart-warming happiness anyone could experience. Finally, some good news and happiness. I couldn't wait to show Christopher. He is going to be walking on air with excitement when he finds out that he has as a baby sister to look after. Oh boy, I know he will be so proud of her.

The whole street is going to know about Claire before I'm even home. Life right now is perfect. A brave boy, a beautiful new baby girl, and a husband (even if he's not so great in the delivery room) is perfect for us all at home. He has promised to protect us and look after us forever.

I simply can't believe the difference between the two birth experiences. But my heart already feels full of love and contentment. All the worries about how to love two children faded away as soon as they passed my perfectly formed beautiful baby girl into my arms.

The look of sheer fear, on the face of Joe will be forever etched upon my mind. My tears of joy flowed relentlessly. I felt so overwhelmed and exhausted once the baby had settled after her first feed that Joe was asked to leave to give Claire and me space to bond and rest. And rest I did! Thankfully, Claire was taken to the nursery for a few hours while I recovered from the ordeal of labour and birth.

A little explanation - Chris is in da house

I hope you're enjoying the book so far. I thought it was the best way of showing the real emotions and feelings surrounding my story. I did this by asking Mum to tell my story through her eyes until I could use my own memories and of the situation. Mum has been there beside me every step of the way. Writing my story this way has meant I was able to allow you, the reader, to follow my life journey chronologically and get a real understanding of the twists and turns my life has taken, allowing your own emotions to carry you along my cobbled path.

Writing the first part of my book from my Mum's point of view gave me a new appreciation of all the sleepless nights she had endured. My medical needs have had a profound impact on Mum and the extended family. After all, I would not have made it this far without their unconditional support. Thanks again, Mum, but I think I can take it from here.

Cue the sarcasm and humour as you buckle in while riding the roller coaster of my journey. I will carry you alongside me while I explain my thoughts and explore the reasons behind them. I will always be as honest as I can, though for those of you embarking on a similar journey, I want you all to realise you're not alone. Every one of our journeys is different, despite being laced with similarities. I just hoped to give you a real insight into life, through the eyes of a transplant patient and all that it encompasses, allowing you to walk with me along the road of discovery and trepidation.

I will endeavour to give you facts and use the terminology that may become familiar to you. A real insight into all the thrills and spills.

There are many spills, especially of my urine as it seeps from the bag that was supposed to be containing it. Oh sorry, did I not give you a warning I was going to talk about the messy stuff. If you're squeamish, please put the book to one side before you ruin the pages. I have spent a while writing this! Other spills to look forward to are the spills of my heart and my mental health.

You didn't think I went through all of this without becoming hurt, disappointed, sarcastic, anxious? At some points I myself was worried about my well-being after reading this. Don't worry, I can see another doctor, I could pop another pill, maybe I could even write a book: oh yeah, that's what I was doing - writing a book.

So, where did my mum get to? Oh yes, a few years have passed, and my cute baby sister had started annoying the hell out of me, constantly wanting to be wherever I was. She always seemed to stick her nose in, even when things didn't concern her. Don't get me wrong, I used to get my own back. After all, I am a blue-eyed boy who could do nothing wrong, especially in my Mum's eyes. That said though, Claire and I were extremely close, she always looked out for me and protected me.

I love her to bits, but I'm never going to admit that. Oh damn, there I go again, messing up as I admit it to the world. Never mind, Claire and Mum know I'm eternally grateful for their support and love. Mum, Claire, and I spent most of the time as a little group, like the Three Amigos.

Anyway, this is my voice from now on.

CHAPTER 7

To Drain or not to Drain?

The weekend had started like those of the past. Mum and Joe had taken Claire and me to Bolton water park for the day. I am now around 8 years old, and Claire is around 4 years old. I vaguely remember that Claire had already started nursery by then.

My fond memories recall a fantastic day full of fun and laughter. The giggles and antics of Claire and I kept Mum and Joe entertained all day. Our day was filled with water park fun. The weather was warm with the sunshine bright in the sky. The bluest sky for as far as my eyes could see. The only shade was provided by the peak of my baseball cap. It was a busy day at the park. There were striped deckchairs in rows along the refreshing waterside, all occupied by adults scantily dressed to absorb as many sun rays as possible. A lot of the dads wore shorts while their t-shirts were tossed over one shoulder accompanied by white socks halfway up their legs and a pair of the brightest white trainers. How cool they all thought they looked. My Mum was relaxed and enjoying some time with her complete family. Mum was wearing a pair of denim culottes, a mix between a floaty skirt and shorts teamed with a pale blue and white, wide-striped tank top.

The fun lasted for ages, playing with friends that were made at the park. Claire and I made up games and challenged each other to do the next daft thing. Oh, how I remember the atmosphere at the poolside! The chitter-chatter of adults filling the air. Then the sound of children squealing with excitement filling the air. The odd raised voice as a parent calls to their child, checking that they were safe or signalling time was up and now it's time to go home.

As I raced through the moving water, I felt a strange sensation in my tummy. I ignored it at first. I distracted my mind with the pile of toys next to an abandoned tower. I waited for a while, checking to see if anyone claimed the toys before I knelt to play with them. Buckets, spades, boats, cars, but more importantly there were two balls. One the size of a tennis ball, luscious green and made of foam. It looked like one of the children had been a bit peckish, a young child-mouth sized piece missing from the foam. It didn't change the use of it though. The other ball, slightly bigger in circumference than a standard football, was inflated by a small plug in the top. The ball had segments of orange and black.

"Christopher!" I heard Mum shout.

My head turned to find Mum in the sea of adults and children before me. Claire was sitting next to me on the floor playing with a select group of girls around a similar age to her. I waved back at Mum. Again, at that moment the pain in my stomach appeared. I tapped Claire on the head and told her I was going to Mum but would be back in a minute. I knew Claire was busy as she didn't even flinch when I touched her head. She didn't move to follow me to Mum either.

When I finally reached Mum, I told her that my stomach was hurting. She shot me a quick response: "You're possibly hungry, it is lunchtime. I will get Joe to go get something from the kiosk soon. Off you go!"

The kiosk was busy. The sign on top of it said open, but I hadn't noticed anyone move forward in the queue for quite a while. The queue of adults and impatient children snaked between the rows of deckchairs. Hopefully, Joe would get some food soon. My stomach was beginning to hurt now.

Joe mentioned that the café may be quicker for us to get some food. Mum asked me to go collect Claire, come back to get dry so we could try the café.

Claire was happily playing with the collection of friends gathered in the same area, though thankfully she was thirsty and took my hand. We walked together to the other side of the park. Mum and Joe were gathering our things together.

Claire and I were already arguing over what we were going to carry to the café, nothing new there.

Claire always found ways to annoy me. She would just shoot me a look or say something and I would want to shout at her. Mum always overlooked the stuff that I did wrong though, so Claire would get told off. Joe, however, knew that I was no angel.

My tummy was getting quite painful by now and Mum was adamant I needed food, she even mentioned having a go on the toilet. I knew I did not need the loo, I'm not a baby. As we arrived at the café my first thought was 'yuck', it smelt like Grandma's chip pan, especially when she needed to change the oil. I gulped as we entered the seating area not sure of the feelings in my tummy. Was I going to be sick, was I going to pass out or was I going to poop my pants? The pains in my tummy got stronger. I told Mum how much it hurt. Once again, her reply was to wait for the food.

That said the food arrived. Claire had spam fritters and chunky chips with baked beans on the side. Joe was served the biggest burger I had ever seen, stuffed with bacon, cheese, salad with browned edges, and a tomato slice that had seen better days. His plate also overflowed with the same oil-slicked chunky chips that Claire had on her plate. Mum had ordered a jacket potato with butter and a side salad. Mum was on one of her everlasting diets. You know the kind that start Monday, but which Monday no one knows.

My plate arrived moments later with a sandwich that again had seen better days. The corners were dried and curled up. The filling of jam was spread so thinly that you needed a magnifying glass to find it. I had a packet of Quavers on the side, though I think the chef got peckish while preparing my lunch. The packet was already open and half the contents missing. I didn't mind as I had no chance of eating. The feelings in my tummy were hurting so much they almost brought me to tears.

I took a small bite of the sandwich, chewing it and moving it from one side of my mouth to the other. When Mum looked over, I attempted to swallow but felt sick. My mouth began to fill with saliva and heat rose throughout my body. My hands became clammy and sweat appeared on my forehead. I took a sip of my chocolate milk, though by now I knew something was not right.

My anxiety kicked in. I sat quietly trying not to be a pest to Mum and Joe. After all, we didn't get out very often as a family for days like this. As soon as Claire had finished her food, I tapped Mum's arm, and at that moment Mum knew I was not well.

Mum told Joe that we needed to get home and that I needed to get some rest. She described me as looking peaky. We left and made for the car. Joe packed the boot while Mum fasted Claire's car seat and I hopped into the back seat. The pain grew more and more intense as we travelled from the waterpark to home.

The journey took around twenty minutes, which is not a long time unless you're in pain, as I was. The car swayed between the traffic and through the build-up of cars across the town. Mum kept looking over her shoulder, checking on Claire and me.

Soon enough, Joe parked the car as close to home as he could. It was just a few metres down from our front door but felt as if I had to climb a mountain. The dread could be seen upon my face.

Mum released Claire from her car seat and barked orders to me: "Get yourself up to your bedroom, you need rest, I will bring you some Calpol once your settled". It was around 2.20 pm when we got home. Claire was disappointed that we had to go home.

So was I, but more importantly Mum was worried as to why I was feeling ill. I overheard Joe and Mum discussing what could be wrong with me and I heard Joe suggest that Mum should call an ambulance. That's when I started to panic. Ambulances mean one thing: hospital.

I have spent enough time in hospital. It's not my favourite place, especially when the weather is so nice outside, and Joe was at home. We should be enjoying days out and visiting friends and family.

Mum was up and down the stairs so often that Joe joked she was wearing out the new carpet thread. Mum laughed and told him to "shut up, something's not right here". Joe met Mum at the top of the stairs and by now I was rolling around on the bed hunched up in pain. I couldn't find a comfortable position. It felt like my stomach was being torn from my body and I was so full it was close to bursting, yet I couldn't go to the toilet. My heart rate was speeding up and my breathing was becoming too fast. My face was flushed red like beetroot, my eyes were swollen and glassy. Mum had reached her limit. By four o'clock she called the ambulance.

Mum told the paramedic all about my medical history. The paramedic was stunned by my history and decided to take me straight to Pendlebury Hospital. They did not want to take any chances. The paramedics radioed through to the hospital and asked for a medical team to be on standby ready to receive me. I had never been in an ambulance before. It was scary.

The paramedic picked me up and placed me on a trolley bed and rolled me into the ambulance. They hooked me up to all kinds of paraphernalia. Mum was grabbing some of our belongings and gave Joe some instructions on what to do next and who to call. She grabbed our bags and the red leather purse that Joe had brought for her birthday.

She knocked on the back doors of the ambulance and without hesitation, the ambulance was moving. I remember the paramedic driving shouted through to the back: "ETA five minutes!"

I recall the paramedic in the back was called David. David was talking to Mum asking her questions about our activities today and what I had eaten. He wrote the answers on a note pad. I was busy looking at all the equipment in the ambulance and wondering what they were all for. I had a monitor on my finger reading my pulse. David also took my temperature and listened to my heart using a stethoscope.

We arrived at Pendlebury Hospital and made our way to Wrigley Ward. All my usual doctors were there and a few nurses. I felt like someone special, if only it had been in better circumstances. The pain in my tummy was now agonising.

The doctor greeted Mum with a smile and said that it hadn't taken long. I didn't know that Mum had previously contacted the ward to ask for some advice. She had already updated them with all the details over the phone and it was the doctor who suggested she should call an ambulance.

The paramedics detailed all their findings to the doctor while the nurses settled me onto a bed in the cubicle. I recognised one of the nurses from my last visit. She was truly kind and was joking with me. She said, "next time you don't want to go on a day out with family there are better ways of dealing with it!" I was in too much pain to laugh. I just lay there until the next pain and I pounced up and got myself into all kinds of shapes trying to ease the pain. I even started crying which I didn't normally do. That pain was far worse than anything I had experienced previously.

The nurses commenced their observations. The doctor then started his normal prodding and poking at me, examining my tummy area. The decision was made to order blood tests before he rang the ultra-sound department and arranged an urgent scan of my kidney and transplant area. He also scanned my bladder and liver, just as a precaution.

Days passed and my results started coming back. The pain was managed by the drip in my arm, pumping painkillers into my body. A steady flow of drugs and observations filled my days and hours.

My consultant arranged for me to undergo a biopsy on my kidneys to test their functioning. My bladder also seemed to be causing concern. Further tests were done on my bladder, testing pressure and capacity.

Mum did not stay in hospital with me this time as she had Claire to look after. Things were a little different when she had more than one child to think about. Mum had to decide which other family members would look after Claire at times because Joe was due to go back to work at this time.

After I had been in hospital for roughly a fortnight the pain was still troublesome, so my consultant took me to the operating theatre to remove my kidney. He was hopeful that the procedure would have eliminated my discomfort and pain. Unfortunately, the pain did not stop. Back to the theatre I went again. They removed my second kidney, only leaving my transplanted kidney to work on its own.

I was beginning to feel like a pin cushion or voodoo doll as I was being prodded and poked constantly. Doctors, nurses, specialists, and even students all coming in and out of my cubicle, all staring at me and reading my notes. Some would even ask if they could feel my painful area. Most would just carry on talking to their teacher while pulling up my top and examining my painful tummy. I would just lay there thinking: "Hello, I am part of this body you know". Everyone would talk about me as if I was invisible.

The adults would make decisions that they believed were the best for me. I would get told things like "it's nothing to worry about", or "let's get you into the wheelchair and get some more pictures of your tummy", always talking to me like a baby. I have spent most of my life in and out of the hospital. I had picked up so much of their lingo and their jargon. Sometimes adults treat children like idiots. *Note to all professionals: children also want to know what's going on and why.*

After a few more days all the attention had turned to my bladder. I went through bladder flushes and even more tests, the daily routines of scans, blood tests, urine tests and observations.

I had nurses checking all my bodily functions. More embarrassingly, a nurse wanted me to do a number two in a cardboard toilet pan, so the doctors could examine that. Is there no privacy or decorum? I had been in the hospital roughly a month by that time.

My parents had got used to daily updates and weekly meetings with doctors and specialists on my progress, or lack of it. The meetings were in place to keep my parents up to date with the findings of all the tests I was going through, and they discussed possible interventions or procedures.

'Options' is a word I learned to dread. Although I knew they were in place to inform, 'options' inevitably meant more prodding and poking, experiments, and operations. Which meant more time in hospital and more tests to be undertaken.

Mum always relayed to me as much information as she could remember.

After all, it's my body that everyone else has a say about, she would say. Everyone had a say except for the one person directly involved. The decisions that were made would impact on my wellbeing for potentially the rest of my life.

Option one: enlarge my bladder and I would have to self-catheterise (self-drain) up to 4 times a day for the rest of my life. I would have to be trained on how to do this, along with Mum as she would be trained too, due to my age. All of this we would have to master before I was able to leave the hospital.

Option two: the surgeon would make a urostomy by using the tissues from my appendix. I would also need a stoma created to attach the urostomy bag to. The bag would act as an artificial bladder which means I would no longer pass urine in the normal biological way that males do.

Mum explained that the consultant had given her and Dad only twenty-four hours to decide. He also suggested that each passing hour gave potential for more damage to my failing organs.

Twenty-four hours passed, well, twenty-six hours actually, and 32 minutes, but that's just me being sarcastic - you will get used to that throughout this book.

Anyway, the consultant sauntered through the corridor and didn't seem to be too worried about my condition. My parents decided to go with…(drum roll please) option one.

This procedure was called the Mitrofanoff procedure, also known as the Mitrofanoff Appendi-covesicostomy, which is a surgical procedure in which the appendix is used to create a conduit between the skin surface and the urinary bladder.

In the procedure, the surgeon separates the appendix from its attachment to the cecum, while maintaining its blood supply, then creates an opening at its blind end and washes it clean.

One end is connected by surgical sutures to the urinary bladder, and the other is connected to the skin to form a stoma. Generally, an incision is made into the navel so it may serve as the canal for the catheter.

Urine is typically drained several times a day by use of a catheter inserted into the Mitrofanoff canal.

Their reason for choosing option one, I discovered a little later in life, was due to my being in school and they were trying to save my blushes if my bag was to leak or if I was to have an accident and my bag fall off. They thought they were protecting me from being bullied. So, the decision was to train Mum and me to be able to catheterise my bladder manually. If you're interested, this means I had to stick a thin tube up inside my belly button until urine came out. As you can imagine this itself can be painful.

However, more than that, it was mind-boggling. How I was going to do this at school or out in public without catching infections or getting it wrong. What I do remember is that at the age of eight or nine years old, no decisions made were down to me. No one asked my view either. I was different from every other child at school, this was just another way my body reminded me that I was different.

The surgical team then came into the cubicle and had a chat with my parents. The doctors spoke about possible outcomes and possible issues, but again I was Mr Invisible, or to them I was.

The next day the training began. Mum was first. The nurse asked me to take off my pyjama top. I was thinking oh, goodness, what are they going to do next? The nurse showed Mum the steps and then Mum had a go.

All I could think was: what has my life come to that my Mum had got to start taking me back to the toilet again, treating me like a baby. Someone please shoot me now! The embarrassment and frustration and feelings of shame struck me like a lightning bolt.

My Mum was also showing signs of discomfort with all this, even though she fought not to display it on her face. Her body gave her vulnerability away. The shaking of her fingers while she followed the nurse's instructions step by step. Her face was a delight. A rosy glow coloured her cheeks from the sheer concentration of holding her breath until she saw the urine start to travel along the tube.

The release of pressure within my bladder was quite a pleasurable feeling. After Mum had completed the catheterization and she felt confident, the nurses turned their attention to teaching me the same procedure. I concentrated hard, after all, I wanted to get out of hospital fast and I couldn't until everyone was satisfied that Mum and I were properly trained. "Come on, Simpsy, you can do this!" a voice urged me from within my mind.

After about 5 days and 3 accidents, I finally got the hang of the procedure and felt confident that I was able to cope at home. Another meeting was held, and the decision was made that I could go home. Woohoo!

I thought I had not been able to see Claire much, and Mum looked exhausted juggling looking after Claire and making numerous trips back and forth to the hospital. Mum always did her best to be with me as much as possible, though I knew it was hard while Joe was away with work. Joe was due home again soon thankfully.

I hoped that another spell of normality would resume at home once we are all back together. I don't want to see hospitals again anytime soon, and I knew Mum felt the same.

On the day of discharge from the hospital, it was like a family reunion. Grandad brought Mum and Claire in the car to collect me to save Mum taking me home in a taxi. Grandma was waiting in the car. Claire seemed overly excited to see me and gave me a big squeeze.

I brushed her off, but that's just the way we are. Mum was quick to warn Claire that I needed space and she wasn't to jump on me or pull me around. I would still need time to get better.

Grandad picked up my bags and said, "do you not want to come home son? I would have been waiting by the door if I was you!" I said: "It's not coming home that's scaring me, it's getting in the car with you!" Mum burst out laughing and stroked my hair, like when you soothe the hair on a dog's back. "Good to see you have not lost your sense of humour lad," Grandad said. Mum went to the nurses' desk to tell them we were going home.

The nurse waved over towards me but I just looked away. Claire had a bag of sweets. I asked for one, but Grandad said, "Grandma has yours in the car waiting for you". With that we all left the ward.

Walking along the corridor I noticed that it was being repainted with rainbows and fairies. Claire went and stood next to the wall and the decorator drew around her outline. He said he was going to use it to draw a special fairy. Claire was over the moon.

We all went on to the car park. That's when I spotted Grandma sitting in the passenger seat of Grandad's car. Her smile would brighten any day and will always make me feel happy.

"Hi Grandma, can I have my sweets? Grandad said you were looking after them for me." Grandma asked for the magic word and then muttered, "manners are free, Christopher, even if you have been in hospital, they are still free". I recoiled and sat on the back seat with Claire and Mum while Grandad filled the boot of the car with my belongings.

Soon enough we were racing through the traffic on our way home. Claire and I were giggling so hard that we even made Mum laugh. She made a noise like a hungry pig as she snorted while laughing at us pulling faces at the passing cars.

CHAPTER 8

Florida, Journey of a Lifetime

It was a shock to me and my Mum, but the nursing staff entered me into a draw to win a 'once in a lifetime' holiday for 2 weeks in Florida. I know that Florida is the magical land of Mickey Mouse, Disney princesses and dream castles.

This was an opportunity provided by a television programme of the '90s.

The BBC programme was called 'Hearts of Gold'. It was fronted by charity fundraiser and ChildLine patron, Dame Esther Rantzen. According to the Google searches I have made, 'Hearts of Gold' also had Michael Groth and Carol Smillie as co-presenters. Running from 29 October 1988 to 1996, the program commended members of the public for their good deeds.

People would usually be tricked into appearing on the show via practical jokes. Courageous and kind-hearted members of the public were lured to the studios for the 'Heart of Gold' award.

There was a real sense of humanity and togetherness as Esther herself was an icon of charitable associations. This programme highlighted the hard work that went into helping and supporting children and their families through all sorts of medical conditions. Their bravery was recognised during their fight against any medical interventions or ordeals that they had to overcome every day of their lives.

This programme regularly pulled in over 5 million viewers on a Saturday evening.

I was so shocked when Mum told me I would be going to Disney World, Florida. OMG, I felt sick, the fizzing feeling in my tummy, and the dizziness of excitement in my head! My breath was caught between my lungs and my throat.

The smile that decorated my face was larger than anyone thought possible. Mum was also smiling and giddy, though what she told me next led me to feel a whole range of emotions.

Mum was happy for me to go, but she knew that I would feel apprehensive once she told me: "The only thing about the trip, is that you're going alone. None of us can come with you. You will be sharing the experience with lots of other children with similar difficulties and health problems. You will have a fabulous time. I'm so proud of you!"

Those words rang in my ears for a while. Alone? No Mum to look after me or to tell me what to do. My anxiety started to implode in my tummy. The fizzy feeling turned to the wibbly-wobbly feeling, like the one you feel when you must have yet another injection, or you know you did something wrong and you may get caught out.

I felt sadness and disappointment for Claire and Mum as I know they would enjoy the experience. Even if they did not like flying that's only part of the experience. Not that they or I know what flying feels like: we have never been on a plane.

Fear of the unknown persisted like night draws in on day. The fear builds the closer the date approaches. The night before the flight my fear got so overwhelming that I had a nightmare and felt like telling Mum that I couldn't go. However, the excitement took over. Like, oh man, can you believe I was going to Florida?! Woo-hoo!

The morning arrived. I was tired from lack of sleep, but fuelled by the excitement. I was hyperactive, bouncing around like a bag of jumping jellybeans. I couldn't even eat breakfast, though Mum tried her best. Mum had packed all that I needed. She followed the inventory letter without deviation: medication, clothes, sun cream, spending money, my favourite toy, the list goes on. Grandad and Grandma visited last night bringing sweets and magazines to keep me busy while on the long journey.

I spotted dad's BMW car driving in the distance, then turning into the street. I shouted through to Mum, "Dad's here, come on we need to go, MUM!"

Dad's cars always changed, but they were always BMWs as he used them for work. He worked at a body shop for cars.

From what he says, it's all about panel beating and spraying paint on car parts, but I forget to listen to the boring stuff at times. It never matters that I don't recognise the car anyway. Last time Dad's car was silver, but this car is dark blue, like the clear night sky.

I could tell it was Dad by the way the car sped along the road, swerving and weaving in and out of parked cars. As he screeched to a halt, the car started smoking from the tyres as the brakes begged for mercy. Dad always drives as if he is the getaway driver in some gangster movie, and he believes he has the lead role! "In his dreams," I thought.

Mum rounded the door of the lounge after finally leaving her haven of the kitchen. She pretended she was washing the breakfast dishes and putting on a wash after stripping my bed.

But I know Mum! She was probably staying out of my way, allowing me to get all the excitement out of my system. I can be annoying when excited, even if I do say so myself. My voice goes all squeaky and I lose all aspects of any simple walking motion. I tend to bounce around on my tiptoes, flapping my arms like Tigger from the Winnie the Pooh collections. Mum just gets frustrated, telling me repeatedly to calm down otherwise I will make myself sick.

"But Mum do you know what it's like to be going on an airplane, I'm going to Disney and I get to see what the clouds look like from high in the sky. I can't wait to wave at you when the plane zooms across the sky above our house. Will you be in the garden, Mum? Will you wave back at me?" Mum smiled while rolling her eyes at me. She warned me to calm down while dad was around or he would not take us both to the airport. Mum was too nervous to drive her little car, that is why she asked Dad to drive us.

By this time, Dad had stopped posing for his public, in other words, the neighbours. Mum shrugged her shoulders and made a comment, but I cannot repeat her words. However, that gives you a flavour of the man my Dad truly is. He is a player, he thinks he is God's gift to women, but we will talk more about that later in my journey. Dad finally made his way up the garden path but before he could reach the door, I swung it open with such gusto that it made a dent in the painted wall. I started dragging my bags to the door and Dad made a comment: "All set I see? ".

I just thought to myself, "no thanks to you", but I kept that under wraps. He doesn't need to know my thoughts right now, and I'm not letting anything ruin my excitement, not even Dad and his self-centred ways. He grabbed my suitcase and backpack and tossed them into the extensive boot of the car, while Mum eventually gathered her belongings and fixed her hair.

After all, she was preparing to meet with all the other lucky children and excited parents at the airport, and there may be media and camera crews from the TV show 'Hearts of Gold'.

The drive to the airport was tense between Mum and Dad. Dad kept his eyes fixed on the road ahead while Mum had her head firmly twisted towards the world outside her window. I remember spotting the road signs with a picture of the airplanes on it. I asked the dreaded question all parents experience: "Are we there yet?"

Mum shook her head. Dad was silent. Well at least there were no arguments this way. I see another sign with the picture and a number 7 on it. "Are we here yet?" Mum turned briskly and shook her head, muttering "Ten minutes!" I started feeling my tummy bubble with nervous excitement. I also felt like I needed to pee. "Are we here now?" I ask again.

Dad looked me straight in the eye from his rear-view mirror and said: "Ask again and I will stop the car and you can walk the rest of the way with your bags". Mum shot Dad a look as if to say, "I dare you...you will be in big trouble!" I sat in silence for the next few minutes until we arrived at the airport.

Now we were at Manchester Airport, I was surprised to be greeted by one of my favourite nurses. She had long brown hair and a smile that lit up a room, like the beam of sunshine that she is. I thought she was there to wish me good luck and have a good time.

Then I was shocked as she announced she had been nominated by the hospital to be the one to look after all my medical needs while we were away. I gave her a hug and Mum smiled. "Surprise!" Mum said. Mum already knew that Edina was the nurse nominated to escort me to Florida. It made then sense why Mum was so calm about my adventures. Mum got on well with Edina and she trusted her implicitly.

There was lots of noise and children. There was an atmosphere of trepidation, fear, anxiety, and excitement and that was mainly from the parents. Some of the children were too sick to be jumping around, though the others made up for it. This would be the first time some children, including me, had been on a flight or left their parents apart from times in hospital. For most of us hospitals were more like our homes and extended families than our actual home.

The process of checking in and having our bags weighed was mesmerising to me. I thought it was magical to put my suitcase onto a conveyor belt and then, whoosh, it was gone. I never saw it again until I landed safely in Orlando Florida.

A part of me thought that all the children had to sit one by one on that very same conveyor belt to get onto the plane. Thank goodness that wasn't actually the way to enter the plane. We did, however, have to walk what felt like miles. I thought to myself, are we bloody walking all the way over there? Why did the plane not park closer? All the parents were waving and crying at the departure gate.

I turned to Mum and saw her big smile, showing her pearly whites. Her arm bore a blouse with capped sleeves and she was waving as if she was the one bringing in the next plane. Dad was standing towards the back of the crowd of parents and a quick nod was the best I got from him.

The flight was so noisy, full of jet blasters, engine noise, and excited children, all of them shouting and screaming. They were fuelled by the sugar rush from the candy-filled bags. Halfway through the flight some of the children got the chance to meet the pilot.

What an experience though! I couldn't believe how many knobs and buttons, shifters and levers there were, with lights flashing and alarms sounding. It reminded me of all the machines and equipment on the hospital wards, though I was amazed at the calm nature of the pilot.

He was very charismatic and exuded kindness. His chiselled chin and piercing blue eyes were set off by a whiff of something expensive that I'm sure would have the hearts of all the cabin crew racing.

I noticed Edina's eyes widen and her eyebrows raised when she saw Captain Handsome-to-All. Oh boy, he knew it too, with a sparkling glint in his eye and the white of his teeth glowing beyond his smile.

All these comments aside, Captain Handsome-to-All was endearing and quite accommodating to the children on board. He even played 'I-spy' with us through the onboard intercom, and then he also announced the first person to find a certain landmark would receive a special gift from him personally. This got all the children excited, or rather it focused their excitement. You could tell that all the staff on board this extremely special flight were hand-picked for their attributes and exceptional way with children. One of the cabin crew, called Darren, played tricks on some of us. He was able to pull coins from our ears, and he would do the odd magic trick as he passed along the aisle checking we were comfortable and topping up our water. It was such a memorable flight.

Captain Handsome-to-All announced that we had reached our destination via the inflight intercom. The seatbelt light above our seats became illuminated, and the cabin crew started their pre-landing checks. The checks consisted of the crew walking from one end of the airplane to the other, moving their beautifully crafted heads from side to side. They reminded us all to put on our seatbelts and return to our selected seats, putting away any loose baggage.

They also handed out hard-boiled sweets to everyone. They said this would help with the pressure change in the fuselage during landing, hopefully reducing the effects on our hearing. The thing that people always complain about after flying is the pain in their ears, or their ears popping. Edina was sitting next to me. She checked my seatbelt was secure, then turned to me and asked if I was feeling ok. I nodded. She then grabbed hold of my hand and whispered to me, "please hold my hand, I am so scared of the landing part!" I laughed at her but allowed her to hold my hand. I noticed her fingers were long and slim, finished with a subtle blush of pink, delicately painted upon each fingernail.

She grabbed hold of my hand so tightly that her knuckles were almost luminous. As I glanced up towards her face, her olive-coloured sun-kissed skin was becoming clammy and her cheeks were glistening, decorated as they were with a shade of rouge.

Edina was dressed in a shift dress with a floral design. Her hair was pinned back sleekly in a high ponytail fixed with a dazzling jewelled clip and an Alice band holding back the stray hairs from her face. Her feet slid into a pair of white plimsolls.

I thought they were her theatre shoes when I first spotted them. Maybe that was my mind playing tricks on me as that is all the nurses ever wear at the hospital. It was quite weird to see my nurse dressed like a non-hospital person.

I know they are people, but I have only ever seen them dressed in their uniforms with watches hanging from their left breast area.

Suddenly I heard the engine noise change. It became so much louder. The sensation of falling from the sky also startled me, as the airplane began to bank to one side, spiralling downwards, though controlled of course. However, this was my first experience and it felt mighty nerve-twitchingly exciting but oh so scary. Then the undercarriage dropped from the underbelly of the fuselage.

My heart started racing and I could feel my ears popping: the kind of feeling when you go underwater and the liquid drowns your ear canals. I tend to hold my nose and try to blow out my cheeks, looking like a chipmunk.

I looked across towards the window and all I could see were the torrential downfalls swooshing past the window. OMG, this was not the Florida I had in mind! Was there a different place called Florida and I had got them mixed up?

When I thought of Florida, I pictured palm trees, scorching sunshine, and vast amounts of highways with all the thrills and spills of the theme parks and wildlife and food so big that one burger could feed a family of four. When we landed it was not anything like the Florida you see on television. We had landed right in the middle of a thunderstorm. Bloody typical, I thought! Just my luck.

We were all piling off the airplane and leaving behind our inhibitions, though I could sense a lot of the children and adults alike were tiring. A good sleep was in order. All the children formed orderly queues along each of the passageways.

The cabin crew, suited and booted looking and smelling as fresh as daisies in a summer meadow, stood to attention at each exit of the airplane. Even Captain Handsome-to-All (so he thinks) graced us with his presence. He could have also been making sure each one of us sugar-rushed kids vacated his vehicle. We were soon all walking along a tunnel fixed to the exit of the airplane.

The tunnel was echoing, each footstep sounding more like a herd of elephants stampeding the savannah. Two well-known Disney characters, Mickey and Minnie Mouse, welcomed us at the other end. Children were screaming and shouting, and adults were taking pictures with wind-up cameras, mementos of their experiences and tales to tell back home.

Once we were all through passport control, we were assigned our tour guides, then directed towards a large double-decker coach with a banner stretching its entire length. This said: "Welcome Children of Hearts of Gold". Advertising at its best for the charity and TV programme that had sponsored us all on this trip of a lifetime.

We finally reached our home for the week. A spectacular hotel, full of all the mod-cons and full of smiles. Every person that passed you had a full smile plastered across their face. The kind of smile that only sinister characters in scary movies tend to wear just before they do a bad deed. However, I believe these people were just in awe like the rest of us at how amazing this place is. Men dressed like Christmas soldiers or drummer boys escorted us to our rooms, bringing with them trolleys filled with our luggage. In the rooms, we got settled, decided on which bed we were taking, and checked out the views from our windows. Finally, a glimpse of the Florida I had dreamed of! Palm trees and, more importantly, there in all its glory: the highest roller coaster bursting through the horizon. The theme park of all theme parks, plus the Disney princess castle stunningly pink with spotlights highlighting its beauty. My heart skipped a beat.

On the first morning we visited an American diner with the freedom to order whatever we liked. I recall ordering my favourite pancakes, of course, washed down with a milkshake. I was amazed at the portion sizes. The glass of milkshake was more like the jug that was placed in the centre of the table back home so that everyone could help themselves.

The pancakes were the size of the steering wheel of Dad's BMW. And there were four or five piled on top of each other, drizzled with maple syrup and chocolate sauce. All of this was for breakfast. These pancakes could have filled a baby elephant. I felt guilty when they were served as straight-away I knew there was no chance I was going to be able to eat these.

That afternoon everyone was frolicking in a huge hotel pool. Groups were introduced to each other and we started sharing stories about why we were there. The hot topic of conversation though was where everyone wanted to visit the most. I was quite reserved and quiet.

I know! Shocking, right, I hear you say! Honestly, my shyness and social insecurities have been debilitating throughout my life.
Hey, at least I have a life, for now.

The following morning, after breakfast, we were all ushered onto the coach for our daily activity. Universal Studios was the destination of the day, with fun and amazing memories to be cherished. Universal Studios was a fantastic experience. We got to watch all the shows and to experience the thrilling rides.

The second day we went to the NASA space station. We got to experience space travel and orbiting. Ok, so not for real, but gosh it felt like it! I found this was the most interesting visit that was scheduled. Learning about all the technology and spacecraft, I was overwhelmed by all the sights and experiences. I found myself daydreaming of travelling to the moon and reaching the stars. Seeing the spacesuits and all the Nasa paraphernalia made me feel like an explorer.

That evening we were relaxing and getting to know each other while enjoying a big summer BBQ accompanied by a disco and karaoke. Children thinking that they were the next famous pop star belting out Spice Girl songs and Kylie's hit, 'I Should Be So Lucky'. One of the adults was showing the kids how to move on the dancefloor. Well, so he thought!

He looked more like a jelly wobbling across the dancefloor with the odd shimmy and shake if you were lucky. He even threw in a high kick and thrust, thinking he was the late great Michael Jackson moonwalking along. I recall the 'Macarena' and 'Saturday Night' by Whigfield being played.

Children and adults showed their fun sides as the Disney characters poured in to give that extra special touch. Now when I look back at these memories, I cannot stop the smiles and my cheeks blush when I think of how I tried to copy the cool kid with his moves. There is always a cool kid. I'm never the cool kid, but I am the kid that everyone wanted to talk to, even when I thought no one had noticed that I slipped off to get a breather. Two girls came towards me asking where I was skulking off to. My fail-safe answer: the loo, obviously. They both giggled as I was heading towards the Ladies. Typical me, getting things wrong or being caught.

We spent our last two full days of the trip we enthralled in the headrush heights of Disney World and Sea World, standing in front of the magnificent Cinderella Castle. The intricate detail of the architecture. The statue of Walt Disney himself opposite. The gardens blooming in colourful flowers. My senses in overdrive.

Edina took my picture standing at the foot of the castle and then we made our way to an ice-cream parlour. After eating the most flavoursome ice cream ever, we made our way to the rides. First, we took a ride on Dumbo, then the magic carpets of Aladdin and on to the river rapids.

My heart skipped as I felt so alive and happy. For once my life was not filled with drug lists and tests, appointments and the regimes of medical stuff. This trip was filled end to end with fun and experiences.

I had such an amazing time. I was so thankful to the nurses for nominating me, but how will I ever repay them. Even so, I knew my happiness and laid-back living would crash down to earth and be smashed to reality once we got back to the UK. This was kind of the way my life goes. No pleasure without pain. If I was enjoying so much pleasure and fun now, God help the pain coming my way.

CHAPTER 9

Experiencing Dialysis

After the fantastic time I experienced in Florida. I was waiting for the bad stuff to come calling. The wait was not that long as, by the age of 12, only 14 months after Florida, I was having to experience the scary, daunting world of dialysis. I should feel lucky, but I don't. Instead, I feel terrified at the idea of undergoing even more procedures to keep me alive. The thought of my body failing me once again cannot be explained in words, though I will try my best. I feel the injustice of my failing health. Why me again? I should be enjoying playing out with my friends or causing havoc to my parents, but I'm unable to have friends round or even attend school regularly like others my age.

The world of renal failure is socially isolating along with the implications for all other aspects of my life, such as my mental health and self-esteem. The idea of dialysis is like when you're having one of those dreams when you see the sunshine and you can hear the sea lapping on the shore, you can almost feel the sand between your toes. Yet, there's a brick wall so high in front of you that there's no way of getting over it. The pure pleasure and sense of freedom: so close and yet so far.

However, the idea of dialysis is to keep me alive until a transplant becomes available, no matter how long that may take. Dialysis is like giving me a rope ladder to help me climb over that wall. It will help me to reach my goal, though it is going to take hard work and determination to get there. It's not going to be easy. I should be grateful, but the dreaded feeling in my stomach reaches its large hand around my throat, restricting my airways, metaphorically speaking.

I know what you may be thinking! I should feel blessed. But I want you to remember that I am not a novice at all these hospital visits, and I'm stuck in here again, hooked up to a machine. That machine is doing the job that my body is unable to complete. I have already had two transplants, which is more than most get a chance at, which I'm more than aware of, though that doesn't mean that I must be happy about going through it again.

Due to my age, I didn't even get a chance to make the decisions that affect my life, which at times can be quite frustrating.

After being given all the advice available at the time, my parents decided to pick the peritoneal dialysis (PD) for me.

My Mum explained that her choice was down to the consultant. He told her that in the world of end-stage renal disease (ESRD) the road less travelled is peritoneal dialysis, though PD is more frequently suggested for younger patients.

This was due to younger patients being more independent and having a better success rate. PD uses osmotic and oncotic pressure, using a machine to place a clear fluid, called a dialysate, into my stomach through a tube known as a catheter into the peritoneal cavity. This fluid absorbs waste products from the blood and then it's drawn back out of the body and discarded.

The ultimate goal of PD is the cleansing of toxins from the blood, normalizing blood electrolyte concentrations, and removing extracellular volume. There are unique complications with PD that relate to the dialytic mechanism itself, for example, peritonitis and weight gain, which are quite common. This is the situation that I was again unlucky enough to find myself in.

I can only recall using this procedure twice, maybe at a push three times, due to the machine filling my body with fluid but not draining it back out of me.

This type of dialysis was usually preferred back when I first learned about this whole new world because it gave people a sense of freedom to continue their everyday lives, where possible.

The medical team decided that the best option for me now would be to switch to using Haemodialysis (HD). HD removes fluid using hydrostatic pressure. This was a machine that I would be connected to by a central line (catheter). The catheter was placed in my neck as an emergency procedure to remove the excess fluid from my body, though I eventually ended up with a permanent catheter in my chest. This meant I was able to go home.

There was an expectation for me to go to the hospital three times a week for up to 5-6 hours a day. I was connected to the dialysis machine for around 4 hours, then I had to add an extra hour for the staff to put me on and off the machine, making sure all the equipment was fully sterile and that my infection levels were stable. I recall visiting the hospital Mondays, Wednesdays, and Friday afternoons.

I would arrive at the hospital at around 12 noon and be ready to be collected by my parents at around 6 pm. I missed roughly 6 hours of school a week. This doesn't seem much time now, but it did affect my confidence in my school abilities and disrupted my friendships.

The hospital had a school on site and they arranged for a teacher to come and work alongside me on schoolwork that I brought with me to the hospital. The school seemed reluctant to give me work to take to the hospital. I assume it was because they thought I was going through enough, though I can't help feeling it was because they thought it was not worth it as I was so ill.

There was an unspoken sense that I could be dying soon, so why bother.

The teacher from the hospital would compensate and give me lots of workbooks around my age and level to keep me busy, a way of giving me something to focus on I am sure.

The consultant and transplant team explained to me and to family members that they now do 'live donors', meaning that a living person can now donate certain organs.

I can recall my Mum asking around the family if anyone would put themselves forward for testing, making sure she gave them all the information available to make an informed choice. Mum and a few of my uncles got tested. Dad (Kevin) refused, saying he would only do it as a last resort. My Mum felt awful that she was unfortunately 'incompatible', which broke her heart.

She would constantly say sorry and tell me how she felt like a failed mother to be unable to help me when I needed it most.

As if she had not done enough for me with all the hospital visits and appointments, let alone cooking and cleaning, sorting schools and all the other paraphernalia of being my Mum.

I tried to reassure her I was not disappointed in her at all. The very fact she even put herself forward to be tested had shown me how brave and courageous she was. Mum is like a warrior in my eyes and always will be. She never stopped her mission to save my life, no matter to what the detriment to hers. My uncles passed the first few compatibility tests, though the further through the process the fewer tests they passed.

This was extremely frustrating for the family, though I had mixed feelings about it. I was fortunate to only experience HD for 6 months. After all the testing and all the hiccups along the way, I received the call. One that was most surprising.

CHAPTER 10

Third Time Lucky?

The call came on a sunny evening in July.

I remember being outside with my friends when suddenly Mum came running, saying "Chris, you need to come home now!" Me being a typical kid, I had to ask her why. Mum then shouted out with an excited voice, though it was tinged with apprehension. As she shouted from the backdoor across the street in the direction I was playing, her words flew from her lips: "the hospital have just rung - we need to get your stuff together and get there as soon as possible, they have a possible match!"

My head started spinning with all the agitation that encompasses yet another kidney transplant. My thoughts cascade between my ears and travel through my body. The involuntary shaking of my anxiety was visible to my friends. They all come running towards me wishing me well and asking questions. The world around me suddenly became noisy with hustle and bustle while I stood frozen as the quizzing of my friends got louder and louder. My body felt as if taken over by robots that carried me towards our back yard.

I shot Mum a look and proclaimed, "Mum you can't be serious!" She replied with, "I am being serious, we have roughly five to six hours to be there. They have tests to carry out, and they need to make sure you're able to undergo the operation". I knew at that moment this was my chance and that it had come for a reason. My heart pounded so hard that I could hear it, let alone feel it. Sweat started to collect on my forehead and my palms became clammy. An excited noise which cannot be explained escaped my mouth. I then shouted to my friends, all eagerly waiting in my back yard: "It's time! I have to go to the hospital, don't miss me too much. Oh, and I won that last game. So that makes it 2-3 to me. See you when I get back!" The kids were fuming! We had a pact that if we went away or couldn't play out, then the game was paused. Ha-ha, I thought, this is a long pause!

I ran upstairs and started collecting my belongings to take with me. The magazines from the floor under my bed. Get your mind out of the gutter, I was 12, it is not a porn magazine. Have you seen the size of me? I could still pass for being in the toddler group, let alone be able to buy adult material from the local newsagents? I then pack my pj's and some socks, slippers, and dressing gown. I will not be needing much more, but not forgetting my pride and joy: the Gameboy console that Gran had bought me last Christmas. I may be able to complete Mario's World by the time I get out of the hospital this time.

Bags packed and I say my goodbyes to my room. It is quite a secretive thing that I do. I look back into my room from the doorway and silently take a moment to take in what I have and what I have achieved, thanks to all the people around me, but especially my Mum and Claire.

They both have given me so much care and unconditional love. After taking a moment, I make my way down the stairs towards the kitchen. That's where Mum is standing opposite the sink with the telephone cord stretched the entire length of the kitchen. She was enthusiastically barking instruction to whoever was on the other end of the phone. I interrupt by throwing my bags down onto the terracotta tiled floor. Something clattered loudly and I cringed with anticipation as to what it was that I was going to find broken when I crouched down to investigate in my bag. Phew! It was just the sound of my deodorant can clanging against the tiles.

Mum shot me a look and, covering the mouthpiece of the phone with her hand she asks, "are you ready?" I nod in agreement. Mum then explains to the person on the other end of the phone that we are about to leave. She confirmed it was ok for them to collect Claire and meet us at the hospital, which would save us getting stuck in rush hour traffic on a Friday.

Mum grabbed a bag of belongings for Claire and herself and double-checked that all the appliances were turned off in the kitchen before we left. I opened the front door and began pushing and shoving with Claire. Whichever one of us got to the car first usually rode in the front passenger seat whilst the other got the back seats. The bonus of being in the front seat was not just that you were in the front, it also meant that you got to pick the music that we listen to on the journey. The stakes could not be higher right now. Claire had occupied the front seat for the last three journeys. Today felt like a special reason why she should have allowed me to sit in the front.

I played the sympathy card on her. Her reply was: "For God's sake, Chris, if I gave you things every time you were ill or went to hospital, I would never have anything or go anywhere!" In true gentlemanly style, I allowed Claire to have the front seat. Who am I trying to kid? In true Chris style I pushed Claire so hard that she tripped over and dropped her things, affording me the extra time to get in the front seat and then I continued to look innocent when Mum appeared. Claire got into the back in a huff. Mum scolded

Claire for being grumpy, telling her "sort your attitude out, missus, it is not your brother's fault that we are having to go through all this again. He did not ask to be ill". Claire muttered under her breath, "Yeah, but it's his fault he is a total twat". Luckily Mum did not hear that. The rest of the journey went well considering Mum was driving and it was rush hour in Manchester. Mum was a nervous driver at the best of times. If Grandad Howard was driving, we would be there in no time. "Better to be safe than sorry", Mum would defend her slow, careful driving skills.

Eventually we arrived at Pendlebury Children's Hospital. Along the brightly coloured, welcoming corridors we tread once more.

Claire stopped to admire an updated wall of art made by the children who had entered one of the critical care wards in the last year. It was like a celebration wall, with lots of inspiring messages of courage and thanks along with the odd drawings of doctors who treated the children. One particularly stood out because the face was all painted blue, as if a pen had exploded on the doctor's face. It made me giggle for a moment. "Claire come on," Mum scolded, "you can daydream later. Christopher is on the clock. If we are much later then his chances slip away again and he will have to be hooked up to that blasted dialysis machine for even longer."

Mum's words demonstrated her perplexity and the inconvenience of me being hooked up to the life-lengthening dialysis machine. Mum never really shows the feelings that have consumed her regarding my health challenges. Mum just inwardly worries and paints on her perfect mask of contentment and optimism, which enables us to get through. But I have heard her sobbing late at night, though these moments are never spoken about. The communication between us as a family is quite minimal, though we know we are all loved.

Once we rounded the entrance of the ward I was greeted with the anticipated smiles and cheery faces of the all-too familiar medical team that were like my extended family. I was then directed towards the side cubicle with the blue end wall.

This was the very same cubicle I had occupied for my second transplant all those years ago. The hardest part was not all the examinations or blood tests. I'm so used to all the rigorous tests and scans, re-tests and prodding and poking. On top of all these things is the mountains of questions and small talk. All these things were not as bad as having a dialysis line - having that fitted was like hell.

The worst part of all these procedures is waiting to see if I was the best match. This is just awful. The medical staff do their best to keep you positive through the torture of waiting. Visualise this: it's as if you're lost in the forest and you come across a signpost with lots of different routes but only one of those routes is your chosen pathway. The rest of the routes circle round and bring you right back to the start. Even worse, you're being chased in the fog by the Grim Reaper. Take a second to process that. How would you feel? All the time you have court jesters trying to make you smile and divert your attention while helping you feel at ease.

The court jesters are my idea of portraying the endearing care of the medical staff as they rally to keep up your enthusiasm. That's essential if the results say that the best match was not you this time. I do hope they come back into the room and tell me that I am the best match, as I'm not sure how much dialysis I could take.

Thankfully, all the tests came back, and I was the best match. Now the next hurdle is keeping me focused and upbeat enough to go to the theatre in a few hours time.

This is a scary idea to process when only three hours previously I was having fun with my friends.

Then Edina, the nurse who accompanied me to Florida just over a year ago, popped in to see me. She opened the curtains just enough to squeeze her head through and whispered, "word on the wards is that we are in the presence of trouble in the hospital. As soon as that was mentioned I just knew it had to be you. No one else around here has such a formidable reputation. I had to come and check it out before all the gossip got out of hand and we were overrun with crowds of screaming girls banging on the doors asking to get pictures with you and getting you to sign their school shirts!" She stifled her giggles as I began to blush. I replied "I think you got the wrong curtains, this one is taken by me. I'm not trouble - that's just something the doctors think about me because I keep coming back".

We both smile at each other and Edina puts her thumbs up and says: "Good luck Champ, I will pop back to see you early in the morning. I'm on an early shift, so it will be me tossing your sheets and annoying you. The pleasure, of course, all mine. Have a good sleep and chat tomorrow!" I shyly shoot her a smile and signal for her to go by pointing to the clock. "I will be going soon," Edina presses her hand on Mum's shoulder, giving it an encouraging squeeze. "See you tomorrow, Wendy," says Edina. "Bye, lovely," Mum mutters back.

The sound of trolley wheels rolling along the uneven non-slip surface increased my anxiety levels as it arrived at my cubicle curtains. Everyone dressed in protective masks, gowns, aprons, and gloves to limit the spread of infection. I was draped in my very fashionable hospital gown while awaiting my fate on what felt like a bed of nails.

My skin felt so sensitive, along with my twitching nerves in my body. The nurses were trying their utmost to wind me up, whistling at my pale chicken legs poking out of the bottom of my oversized gown. They didn't care if I was beginning to feel embarrassed or not, they were like family to me, which allows them to taunt and tease me as if I was at home. They say it is all about the character-building of a child. They joke, saying it makes us feel at ease and allows us to feel like we are part of the team. I jump down from the bed and hike myself on to the trolley. Mum passes me a blanket, covering my modesty, though I just wanted this ordeal to be over.

It's strange, the more need for interventions and treatment, the more I feel like I'm a burden to the medical staff, even though they try to joke with me. Sometimes I feel the frustration rising in my veins. I feel like I'm taking the place of others who could be better suited. Yet, at the same time, I'm in complete awe of all the medical staff who have continued to put my every need first, concentrating on my well-being and quality of life. They must see something in me that I don't as yet.

The nursing staff checked everything from paperwork to next of kin, to dietary intake and last drink, to the last time I went to the loo and even the details of colour, consistency and more. There's no privacy when you're a renal patient.

All of this before we embark down the bumpy corridor with all the 'well wishes' splattered between paintings of superheroes and butterflies along the wall to the theatre. Soon I was in the 'sleep room', otherwise known as the anaesthetic room.

The staff were laughing with me, yet again making references to me having a dream date or the next footy championship, all of this while checking my notes. As always, the doctor turned to me to explain everything he was doing step by step. Sometimes I wish they would just get on with it. It's not as if

I can do anything about it anyway. He then turned to Mum saying they were going to put me to sleep in a few minutes. Mum kissed me on the forehead like always, whispering, "see you later, behave in there and I love you!" This was a staple comment Mum would always say to me when I was going under anaesthetic.

This would hopefully allow me to undertake the operation without pain or suffering. I counted backwards from ten. I think I got to 'seven' and I was gone.

The next thing I remember I was being woken up by Edina as promised. The rest I'm unsure of. I knew something had been done because I was feeling groggy and sore. Time for pain killers and drains to be checked. At least I know one thing, I survived yet another operation. More importantly I was given the chance to live by someone who had lost their kidney: a truly heroic act by any standards, for which, regardless of viability or longevity, I will be forever grateful.

CHAPTER 11
GCSE's, Kidney Failure and Haemodialysis

A few years passed, and Mum was no longer married. In total honesty, I'm unsure when she and Joe separated or why, but I know she was not as happy as she allowed others to think she was. She was currently seeing a guy called Paul, from Wrexham in North Wales. Finally, Mum had met a man who was treating her as she had always deserved, in my eyes at least. Paul would do anything he could for Mum, but not just Mum, us kids as well. Claire and I adored him. Mostly due to the way he made Mum feel. He brought out the best in Mum and made us feel like part of a family.

Claire and I found it hard adjusting to life again with Mum and her new fella, but Paul always included us and did his best to make things work between us all.

Claire and I took a while to accept Paul and to get used to Mum having a partner again. After all Mum had been on her own for so long. We had become a formidable force, the three of us. Paul lived with his mother as he was her carer. Paul would just say she is his Mum and it's his role to look after her, after all, she did it for him when he was young, now it's his turn to care for her when needed.

I believe It was around Easter time, if my memory serves me correctly. We were on holiday at Paul's mother's house. During our break in North Wales, I began to get pains in my stomach. Mum and Paul took me to the Maelor Hospital in Wrexham. I was transferred to the children's ward immediately. I was around fifteen years old.

The nurses and doctors at Maelor were lovely, just like those at Pendlebury Hospital, where I had my previous treatment. I distinctly remember one of the nurses who was quite tall, stocky in build with short grey hair and a very calming voice. (I know what you are thinking, anyone would be tall next to me. You may be right, but this nurse was exceptionally tall. I remember thinking, I wonder if he will need to bend down to get through that doorway at the end of the corridor? That kept me amused most of the afternoon, while I waited). I can't remember his name, but I would be able to point him out if I was to see him again. He was lovely, very reassuring and he even cracked a joke or two, though I thought they were badly timed.

I vaguely remember the nurse asking who last cooked and what it was. Mum was not happy at all. She turned to Paul and said, "is he for real, is he accusing me of poisoning my child? Paul laughed and said, "he knows you well then!" Mum was not seeing the funny side at all. The nurse quickly diverted our attention and pointed out areas such as the playroom and a room with tea and coffee facilities for Mum and Paul while they waited for some test results and for a consultant to examine me.

However, soon after the consultant saw me, he explained his conundrum. He needed to discuss my case with my consultant from Pendlebury Hospital. I was moved to the Cunliffe Ward later that evening. Cunliffe Ward specialised in renal cases and urology. I can't remember how long I was there, a few days at most. Then it was decided I should be transferred to Manchester

Royal infirmary. I remember being on a ward at the Infirmary when my lung collapsed. I needed the intervention of a ventilator.

This was extremely scary. All this was new to me and Mum. I had never suffered any breathing difficulties before, apart from being asthmatic, which was well controlled. Now my body seemed to be failing one organ at a time. I had to undergo constant tests and procedures.

I was taught how to breathe again, with the aid of a face mask. It was awful, very exhausting. I managed to get my lung functioning properly again over time, though it never seemed as good as before for many months.

Sometime later, I was transferred to Pendlebury Hospital, placed on the ward I practically grew up on. I was not getting any better. I think by now it was around May because they were preparing an education plan. They were trying to come up with a robust action plan, for me to sit my GCSE exams while being an inpatient.

Anything I ate or drank was not staying where it was intended. I ended up either throwing it up or having chronic diarrhoea. (Sorry for the vivid view but I did say this book was honest and graphic). This was interfering with the antibiotics as my body was rejecting those too. All of this was having a knock-on effect with other aspects of my wellbeing too. I was losing weight constantly which I could not afford to do as I was already on the lower end of the chart for my age. The weight loss and constant sickness were making me so weak. The extremely limited energy I did have in my body was needed to fight to keep me alive. It was decided that I be put on complete bed rest. That meant that the nursing staff had to do all of my care, from washing, dressing, and making my bed to feeding me or helping me to take sips of water from a straw.

I think this was the first time that I honestly believed I was going to die. I began to get scared, thinking this is the end. Nothing the doctors suggested seemed to be working. We are now in June, which was exam time, plus Mum and Paul were getting married next month.

Paul was such a gentleman. He even asked my permission to marry Mum, which was nice. I think for the first time in my life I felt valued by another man. Paul asking me for Mum's hand in marriage made me feel respected, especially as I was the only male left in our family. Up until now it had been just the three of us. I did, however, take this opportunity to warn him, asking if he was sure he wanted to marry Mum. I suggested that he might regret that decision. We both laughed a little and there was some banter between us, but If anyone could stand by Mum and us when we needed him then I think he could.

Paul proposed to Mum on New Year's Eve 2000, at the turn of the Millennium. It was so special and romantic. Paul got down on one knee in front of all Mum's friends. Mum was mortified, she got very embarrassed and after a short pause she looked round to see everyone was expecting her reply. She just shouted: "Yes!" She was overjoyed and burst out crying. Mum was always an emotional wreck and would easily cry over anything. Luckily enough for me I haven't inherited that as it would be awful. I didn't often witness that side of her. Claire didn't either. Mum was very grounded and assertive when it came to her children.

Mum and Paul quickly set a date for the wedding, which was going to be July 2002. This gave them 18 months to save up and prepare us kids. This date was a few weeks after my GCSEs. They had also planned to move to Wrexham together. The move had come as a bit of a shock to Claire and me. I should have been preparing for my GCSE's and Claire had only just started high school. Claire was debating whether she should move in with her dad, Joe. This would afford her the stability of staying at the same high school. Her other option was to move with Mum and start all over again, moving to a new school and making new friends.

I didn't know if I wanted to move with them either, as I was sort of talking to my Dad, Kevin, too. I was also extremely close to my grandparents, who I couldn't imagine having to move away from. Kevin had recently got married in 2000.

Dad and his new wife were expecting a baby in the autumn of 2002. I was unsure of what to do. I had never lived with Dad apart from stopping over for maybe a week or two. That was always enough as we would start arguing by then. So, this was going to take some careful consideration for us all.

One morning, while I was thinking about my decision on whether to relocate to Wrexham with Mum or not, one of the nurses, I think it was Edina, came in and asked me if anyone had tested the water I had been drinking.

I thought that was a dumb question. How do I know what everyone had done and not done, after all, I'm just the one suffering all these things and feeling worse by the minute? All I could focus on was at this rate I'm not going to make Mum's wedding if I don't start to get better, and quickly. I think they had tested and tried everything else. They were running out of options.

The nursing staff decided to test the water I was drinking. It was a surprise to us all: the result from the water tests concluded that it had cryptosporidium in it. Cryptosporidium can cause respiratory and gastro-intestinal infections.

Devastatingly, I also found out that my third transplant had been struggling to cope under the strain caused by the cryptosporidium. My third kidney was now failing. My world yet again spins into a cyclone of tests and more hospital interventions, let alone the thought of the extended periods I would need to be eating hospital grub.

This also meant I would need to be hooked up to Haemodialysis (HD) once again. The idea of going back on HD was not a joyous prospect for me, let alone my family. Mum was so sad, and you could see the real disappointment in her eyes. Even her encouraging and uplifting words betrayed her inner thoughts. My thoughts were far more direct and outspoken. With phrases such as: "Oh for fuck's sake!" "Why me?" "Will I ever get a break?" My darkest thought at that time was: "I give up, just let me die". My body does not want to see adulthood and be a party to all the things that I have dreamt of achieving. I thought perhaps I was being punished for something, though I have no idea what.

The medical staff were not giving up on me just yet, so it looks like I can't either. I need to battle on and find the strength from somewhere. Once the hospital put everyone on bottled water, changes started to appear. They also increased my intravenous (IV) fluid intake and my recovery made great leaps.

I found a nugget of courage. I dug deep to show determination and tenacity, pushing myself through physio. All of which was for my Mum and Paul. I so desperately wanted to walk Mum down the aisle.

I knew that I had to be well enough and build my strength up. Though I was told to concentrate on just being well enough to be able to go to the wedding, anyone who knows me knows that was not enough for me. I had to dig deep here, finding the warrior in me to fight this battle long and hard. I surprised everyone including myself. I don't know how, but I managed to get home and be at the wedding.

I was so proud of myself.

After the wedding and all the celebrations were over it was time to make that big life-changing decision. To move or not to move. Claire decided she wanted to move to Wrexham with Mum and Paul. I didn't blame her as she was only young. It would be easier for her to make a new start. I decided to stay put in Manchester with Dad and my grandparents. I also had the support of my friends in Manchester. Even more of a deciding factor was that I knew the hospital staff and they knew me. I thought that, for now, staying in Manchester would be my safest option even though I was going to miss Mum and Claire immensely. They were only a train ride away if I needed them and we could talk on the phone too. I felt Mum deserved to be happy and have a break from hospitals and from me. She had devoted her life to Claire and me, now it was her time to be loved by Paul.

I made great progress with my health and became quite stable. This allowed me to start planning career paths that I would be interested in pursuing at college. I had decided that Childcare or Health and Social Care would suit me as I had a lot of insight and an invested interest in them. I would like to progress into nursing one day if possible. I applied for both Childcare and Health and Social Care, so I had a fall-back plan, if needed to depend on my final grades.

I was thrilled to be offered interviews for both courses and to be offered a place on either course if I reached the required grades. Fingers crossed, I thought.

CHAPTER 12

Health and Social Care

September arrives with gusto and my education journey picks up from where I left off. My exam results were fantastic and shocked many people, not least my school tutor. She had previously asked me to consider cancelling all of my exams except my core requirements of English, Mathematics and a Science. I knew best though, as always! I sat all of the exams I was entered for. To everyone's astonishment, I passed them all with 'C' Grades or similar, which allowed me to progress to a foundation Health and Social Care course at Bury College.

Things in my life have changed dramatically since I sat my GCSE's back in June. My life journey sounds more like a TV drama than real-life experience. As I sit here listing the main events, even I feel these events are quite dramatic. I can assure you though, they are not exaggerated. In the last six months, I have been exposed to many worrying situations, such as my kidney transplant failing. I needed to recommence the use of my life-machine, the Haemodialysis.

You the reader are now accustomed to my life patterns, or at least beginning to be. My life also had a few occasions to be proud of and to keep me focused on the positive side. My life always follows a pattern of pleasure-pain. My mental health has started to become more troublesome of late. I worry about all aspects of my life. Especially after another failed transplant by the age of 16. These endless operations and doctors' appointments, blood tests, scans, and interventions.

The fact that Mum was so happy to be marrying Paul allowed me some much-needed respite. The burden I secretly feel is that I have to carry on fighting my health demons. To be able to be here for Mum. She never gave up on me, so how could I give up my fight for life?

However, I feel more reassured that Paul will take care of Mum now, allowing me to get on with the job in hand: surviving my life. Mum and Claire moved to Wrexham with Paul. My living arrangements have also taken a different direction. I'm now residing with Dad, his wife, and my adorable, if noisy, baby brother Mathew. Matthew was born on 3rd October 2002. I found that having Mathew around gave me a new zest for life and a sense of purpose.

Life was completely different now. My new world was partly consumed by being hooked up to dialysis, and partly by my role as a full-time student in college. Not forgetting the new baby in the household. Dad's house is big enough and his wife has done her bit to be welcoming, though I understand this was not what she had planned for their newly married life with a new-born.

My days were still filled with the same routine of dialysis. This worked well, so I didn't miss too much college. There must have been an angel looking down on me because the only lesson that I was missing was English on a Wednesday afternoon. I'm not a religious person but if there is such thing as a God, I would press my palms together and say, "Thank the Lord!"

The course helped to keep me motivated and the students were quite accommodating and friendly. Some would even invite me out on our days off. Unfortunately, more often than not I would have to decline their offers, due to me being hooked up to HD or having blood taken or having rest days. I was enjoying being a college student, but it was taking a lot of effort to keep up with deadlines and coursework when at home. I tried to make the most of my flexibility. Learning to be organised was the key to my success.

Inevitably, living with Dad was not what it was cracked up to be, although deep down I always expected it to turn out like this. Dad and I have always had an arduous relationship.

I feel that I put in 80% of the work, while his 20% is made up of saying hello to me if he could be bothered, or transporting me to hospital. He thought that was all it took to be a supportive father.

I don't think fatherhood came naturally to Dad. To make things worse, I felt like I let him down or didn't live up to his expectations most of the time. I think he finds it hard to bond with me. Every time we plan something I end up with an infection or needing a hospital visit.

It must be frustrating for him, yet, try being me! See how I feel about things. He never asks if I'm ok or if I have things under control. Dad just expects me to just get on with it. This is because hospitals and tests have been my whole life since the day I was born. I always felt like an outsider encroaching on his perfect little family. I didn't belong there, and Dad didn't put up a fight at all when I told him how I was thinking and my plans to move to Wrexham to Mum.

Summertime 2003, I moved to Wrexham with Mum, Claire, and Paul. There were many factors that had to be considered. Mum and Paul were happy for me to move in with them. Claire, on the other hand, had been used to having Mum all to herself for a while. I didn't blame her. After all, Claire's life and relationship with Mum have always played second fiddle to me and all my health needs. So, rightly, Claire was always happy to see me, but there was some slight animosity between us.

One of the main reasons I decided to move to Wrexham to was the offer of a preliminary place to do a level 2 Health and Social Care course.

The only stumbling block was that I was expected to do a considerable number of weeks work-based placements to pass the course. It was a requirement from the examining board in order for me to gain the qualification.

After careful consideration, my tutor has shown empathy regarding my health needs. However, she was also very aware of the expectations placed on students on placements. My limitations were now starting to become more apparent. My tutor felt that with my Haemodialysis it may be wise to put my studies on hold.

The certificates I have already would always be worth something, and I could recommence studying when I was feeling better. Yet again, my health was holding me back. Every time I tried to make something of myself, or take a more positive pathway in life, my health or a related issue would stand like a blockade, causing a halt in my life.

These situations are quite frustrating. I get angry about my illness, though I tend to take it out on the people or things surrounding me. I can throw a cup as far as an Olympic standard javelin athlete, and with as much force as Muhammad Ali throwing his last knockout punch against Richard Dunn. Don't get me wrong, I don't hit people, but I have started breaking things more often. I believe I have a lot of pent-up angst about situations out of my control. It doesn't mean I feel things any less though. I resent my body and all its ailments.

I often feel in conflict within my thoughts. The days I feel like giving up are long and difficult to shake off. I usually do this by listening to music. I have used music for a long time to help sooth my inner demons and negative thoughts. Then I think of the people who lost their battle with life, which in turn allows me a to battle again. Hopefully, this will be the fight that I win.

Everyone was flabbergasted, including me, when I achieved a Merit grade in Health and Social Care. Mind you, the self-critic in me was aiming for a Distinction. I had lived and breathed the heady heights of Health and Social Care. If I didn't understand it by now, then I have bigger issues. This meant that I could excel at the next level.

But as I said, my tutor thought it is best that I concentrate on conserving my energy and getting my health to a reasonably stable state. "Good luck with that!" I thought, but I will give it a go. At the end of the summer term, I started to make plans to move to Wrexham with Mum, Clare, and Paul.

CHAPTER 13

Moving to Wrexham

Living with mum, Paul and Claire was once again a completely new experience for me. It was a little difficult for me to adjust at first. I was practically a stranger in a new town. I didn't know anyone. I wasn't as confident or vocal as Claire, who made friends easily. She was outgoing and confident whereas I was shy and self-conscious, constantly worried about contracting an infection or needing yet another hospital visit.

I first met my new renal consultant in what I would call a welcome meeting. I had a walk around the unit and was introduced to the renal team that would be taking over my care while I resided in Wrexham. I found this all very formal and professional, not at all like what I was used to at Pendlebury. Maybe because at Pendlebury they were more like my extended family, I didn't know any different.

The Maelor was more clinical and more like the kind of unit you would refer to as an adult's unit. After I visited Wrexham Maelor Hospital it dawned on me that I was now moving more towards adult care as I was seventeen years old, potentially classed as an adult patient. I will soon be able to sign my consent forms and make decisions about my health and what I agree and disagree with.

I became quite overwhelmed at the thought of making those decisions. Some of the decisions that Mum has had to make for my care over the years could have gone very wrong. Well, as you can tell from the book so far, some interventions have not always worked out as intended.

My mind started racing and whirling at the very thought of my first decision, which would be my next transplant if I'm lucky enough to make it that far. I quickly shook the negative feelings to one side as Mum shouted my name from the corridor: "Christopher! The doctor asked you a question." My eyes widened, and I apologised to the doctor.

A nurse rounded the corner and instantly I felt a sense of calm. Her smile was warm and friendly. Her stature suggests she is a senior member of staff. This was confirmed as another nurse entered the ward and the older nurse gave the more youthful nurse instructions.

The senior nurse then made her way towards Mum and me, extending her hand after washing at the nearby basin. Her smile was framed with bright pink lip liner. Her smile was so inviting.

Her confidence was apparent in her voice. "You must be Christopher?" she said while taking my hand. I shook her hand and she gave me a cheeky wink. "My name is Julie. I have been studying your medical records and, boy, you are a phenomenon! I bet you feel like a robot with all the procedures you have had."

I smiled shyly. Finally, someone who gets it I thought. I felt comfortable already. Julie then moved her attention to Mum, asking her some questions. I remember Mum laughing. This sticks out in my memory as Mum doesn't laugh like that often. It was a genuine chuckle. Her nose wrinkled and her shoulders rose and fell with each breath. Mum's cheeks started to glow. To this day I don't know what Julie said to Mum, though I will always be thankful that she made her smile. I soon learned that Julie has a special gift.

She can make anyone who encounters her feel at ease and she can make you laugh at the most inappropriate times. I left the unit feeling confident in their care. I felt optimistic I would receive sensitive and personalised treatment.

Even so, I was feeling slightly sad at leaving the familiarity of Pendlebury, especially the staff who I have mentioned previously, such as Edina and others. They were more like family members to me. I spent far more time with them than my actual family. After our look around, Mum and I went home to prepare for my first dialysis session on the adult ward. This was such a different experience for me.

The ward itself was more suited to the needs of an adult, including the magazine rack fixed with gold screws to the wall at the far end of the unit by the entry doors.

There were no more colourful walls with cartoon characters or superheroes. Instead of Superman saving a boy hand painted in all its glory spanning the space across the wall at Pendlebury, the renal unit in the Maelor was painted with generic magnolia, broken up with a broad band of blue painted halfway up the walls. Wrapped like a present tied with a bow at Christmas, all that was missing was the surprise inside. Instead, there were machines, tubes, doctors, and nurses buzzing around, busy with their schedules.

That evening I started dialysis on the adult unit. I didn't know what to expect because I was used to playing games and having fun. In Pendlebury, the nurses would try anything to make the experience of dialysis as enjoyable as possible. When I arrived at the unit with Mum and Paul, a nurse greeted Paul saying, "nice to meet you, please follow me to get your blood pressure and weight done". Paul's face was a picture! He looked so scared, Mum and I were laughing until Mum had to intervene.

"Excuse me," said Mum, "this is Christopher!" She pointed to me while still laughing. The nurse looked mortified and she apologised profusely, saying: "I'm sorry he looks so young!" This was a perfect example of when a nurse talks about you without even acknowledging you. The nurse could have made the same comment, but she could also have spoken to me along the lines of, "gosh, what soap are you using, you look far too young to be here?" A comment like this would have made me giggle and feel included, which might have even made me feel good about myself.

Instead, I instantly felt like I was in the wrong place and that I didn't belong. A misfit once again. Language and communication are so important when conversing with service users or patients.

I followed the nurse to get my weight and blood pressure checked. The nurse then showed me to my allotted seat. This would be my new home for the foreseeable future. I can recall the nurses and other patients looking at me and whispering. "He is so young to have to go on dialysis," was a common statement.

Paul left to do some shopping while I spent time on the machine. Mum stayed with me to keep me company, especially as this was my first time on dialysis here. Mum told me that while I was getting weighed one of the other patients was quizzing her about me. She asked how old I was. The female patient was visibly shocked to learn that I was merely seventeen.

I soon got used to the dialysis unit and the nursing staff. Once again it became just another routine which is in place to extend my life. I think that some of you reading this book can only imagine the extent to which my life has been overwhelmed by routines, injections, appointments and hospital visits, let alone therapy and rehabilitation sessions. Sometimes I look back on my childhood and find myself consumed by jealousy and discontentment. I feel like I missed out on a normal childhood where I could play out in the park for the whole summer or have sleepovers at my friends.

Friends, what are they? I have had very few friends in my life and even the ones I have had have mostly been fleeting, a little like my relationships. Mark is one of the only friends who have stood by me while I have gone through the many procedures needed to help me survive until now. When I think about my future, I get quite fearful, though I never admit this to anyone. I keep a lot of my feelings bottled up inside. I would never want to come across ungrateful for all the support my Mum has given me, along with all the nurses and doctors. But thinking of my future keeps me awake regularly at night.

Once I had turned eighteen, I knew realistically that I couldn't live with Mum and Paul forever. Plus, one day I would like to hopefully have my own little family. Unusually, I felt comfortable enough to open up to one of the dialysis nurses who was sitting with me while I was on the machine.

Julie, the nurse, was so supportive during my sessions. She listened intently and she would reflect some of my words back to me. It was really powerful to have someone repeat the exact words to you.

I started to realise that I was struggling with many issues and that I would need some professional help to start untangling the web of mixed-up thoughts and feelings surrounding my existence. Julie recommended Caron, the renal social worker. She said that she would advise me on the different options regarding benefits, grants, employment, and housing issues.

I had the same worries as everyone else though I just had the added disadvantage of my health to worry about. I was beginning to get itchy feet about living at home with Claire, Mum, and her Paul. I was 19 and still single. This wasn't going to change anytime soon, while I was still living at home.

My routine of doing dialysis three times a week in the evening was keeping me alive. Nevertheless, in my heart I knew that the machine wasn't all I had to live for. I knew that if I was careful and sensible, well, sensible for a nineteen years old single lad, I could live a reasonably normal life. Many people do who have been fortunate enough to be able to use dialysis.

Unfortunately, due to my numerous health issues, it was like a living hell being on dialysis. This was because of my experience of dialysis and being only nineteen. I found it hard in reality.

It's the things we take for granted that matter, like being able to get an interview or apply for jobs, do a fulltime course in college, planning a family event or meeting up with friends. All of these things became almost impossible because I was constantly in and out of the hospital due to infections or access issues.

I couldn't put on my CV that I have never worked since leaving school due to being hooked up to a dialysis machine three times a week. I couldn't mention my susceptibility to infection and that I could end up in and out of the hospital every month. No employer in their right mind would want to offer me a job knowing my limitations.

Discrimination happens in many ways. However, I believe disability discrimination is hard to eradicate, especially where hidden disabilities are concerned.

For instance, if an employer or member of the public was to meet me for the first time, they are most likely to assume that I have nothing wrong. In reality, my body is extremely frail and slowly deteriorating. However, all of this is on the inside and to the unaccustomed eye I look perfectly normal, even if a little on the shorter side of average. No one would suspect I had such a debilitating disability unless you know me.

I would regularly return home after dialysis and go straight upstairs to bed, put my headphones on and quietly cry myself to sleep. This was due to frustration and sadness more than pain. I so desperately wanted to be normal. I wanted to be able to be carefree and lead a typically normal life with a girlfriend and job, my own home and my own family. The older I get the more resentful I become at not having the life I hoped for. Instead, I have to endure the relentless hospital visits, blood tests, appointments, infection control and dialysis.

I know deep down that all the pain, struggles and suffering make me who I am. Just sometimes, even if for a little while, I would want to be normal. Hopefully, one day I will make my children and partner extremely proud of me, if I am blessed to get to that day. But as you know by now, there are always twists and turns in my life and moving to Wrexham was just the beginning of a turbulent roller coaster trail. Are you brave enough to hold on tight and endure the rest of my journey? Surely there are some highs to come if we grin and bear this bit together, I'm sure we can get through the rest. Hold tight, things are going to get a little bumpy!

CHAPTER 14
Love and Heartbreak

Online dating is not for everyone, though if you're in my position it can be the only way of communicating with potential partners. You have the opportunity to get to know each other without my illness being at the forefront of all conversations. It gives me a chance to show the other sides of me. Hopefully, my personality comes through and that is what the ladies will fall in love with, instead of the usual pitying faces when people learn of my illness and struggles. I suppose it gives me a sense of confidence and control to be able to tell the women what I feel comfortable with. I don't have control over my body and mind most of the time due to the necessity of doctors knowing what's best, or my Mum usually making the decisions. Online dating allows me a sense of empowerment and freedom.

I tell potential partners about my health conditions when I feel the time is right, when I decide and not my Mum or a doctor. At least if I'm honest and true to myself then it's easier to be open with potential suitors. There's nothing I would want more than to be able to have some kind of normality in my life, a lady to treat like a princess, someone to love and to receive love from. To have closeness and intimacy, though all of this I would overlook if I could just find someone who could accept me for who I am, my health being part of that.

I first met my partner using the online dating sites I had signed up to. I don't know if this is just me or whether you have noticed that dating as changed over the years. I feel that online dating helps to accommodate the fast pace and challenges of the 21st century. I believe this has been for the better in cases like mine. It alleviates some of the restrictions on where and when I can go out. I acknowledge that many stories are emerging in the press of these dating sites being abused. Like everything these days, there is always a select few misusing a system and ruining it for the masses. Like when someone impersonates different characters, or when past lovers changing their profiles to trap and entice past love interests. I'm sure these were never the intentions of the creators of the dating sites.

I noticed that my health issues had impacted on my confidence levels, which made me feel inferior to others. I felt extremely awkward and shy around new people. I would even start to blush just saying hello, especially to the opposite sex. I feel I missed out on all the practice and socialising skills that most develop during their adolescence in high school and college. I spent my adolescence in hospital and there's not much chance to flirt or romance in those places. Unless you count the nurses winding me up or pulling my leg. Any potential partner that I met were also patients. They would be too wrapped up in their health worries to even be thinking of dating or investing in a relationship. So here I am, giving the keyboard a tinkle and putting my computer skills to the test while I give online dating a whirl. Surely it can't be so bad, after all if I don't like it, I just politely say goodbye and switch off. What's the worst that can happen?

I entered my details and agreed to all the necessary notices and warnings and adhered to the rules. I spent a good few hours reading all the paraphernalia and safety advice attached to the site. I agreed to the terms and conditions and before I knew it

I was creating a profile. OMG, I need to add a picture! I hate my picture being taken at the best of times. Now there's the pressure of finding a picture that I don't look ill, stupid, or tired in. I want to give the right impression without looking desperate or goofy. I want to be taken seriously, though I am fun-loving at heart. Do I add a picture with a smile? Or should I look serious? Do I wear my glasses or no glasses? This was already becoming a whole new world of decision-making with mixed emotions.

I had not even entered the details about my illness or the kind of partner that I'm looking for yet. All this over a bloody picture! Come on, Simpsy, get your act together I thought to myself.

What details do I add to this profile? Then my head started wandering off into the realms of negativity. Thoughts of giving up and succumbing to the fact that I'm destined to be alone all my life. How do you explain to a potential new partner: "Oh, by the way, I have a life-threatening condition which means I have to be attached to a machine three times a week to stay alive." Am I being selfish wanting to be with someone while I'm uncertain of my future?

If the shoe were on the other foot would I even put myself forward and commit myself to someone if they were unsure whether they will still be alive two years from now? This left me pondering and I closed down the site while I decided what to do and how I felt about myself and the idea of allowing someone into my life. The idea of having someone with me and walking along my uncertain path was great, but the reality was far more intimidating than I had thought.

A few days passed, and another dialysis session. I chatted with Julie once more while she was hooking me up to my lifeline. Caron also passed by where I was sitting and before I knew it my love life, or lack of it, was the topic of conversation on the whole unit. I felt embarrassed by the conversation, though I was pleased that I had managed to even open my mouth and ask for advice. Caron and Julie quickly became my champions and supported my attempts to be happy. They did their utmost to make me feel valued and accepted on the unit. They even gave me tips for explaining my illness to people in a more sensitive way. Julie would always joke with me and say, "why do you even need a lady friend anyway when you have such amazing nurses looking after your every whim here?" Her smile is as big as her heart and her warmth as comforting as the cosy blanket I remember being wrapped in as a young child when I was having a sick day on the sofa.

Eventually, I plucked up the courage to complete my profile on the dating sites. After a short while, I started getting requests and messages from beautiful ladies. After a few messages their responses would be the same over and over again. They would say: "You are a nice lad and friendship is all I see between us". This got so repetitive that my ray of the hope for finding a partner began to diminish.

The comments about 'friendship not romance' were the standard reaction. I didn't plan to make friends, I was desperate to have a life partner, someone to share a bucket of popcorn with while sitting on the sofa watching a movie. Someone to stand next to while watching the sea lapping at the shore. Someone to cry with while feeling low, and someone to share my achievements with when I conquer my goals. It's not too much to ask, is it?

I always had the dilemma: do I tell them straight away on a first date? Or do I let them get to know me first? I have had a few dates now and have tried both. In all honesty, the latter option is awful. The experience of getting close to someone, and then their true colours come out after you tell them your health condition. However, I have to take some responsibility for this and I do always ask for honesty in all my relationships, especially friendships. I can't abide fakery and untruths. These are my dating experiences, and I am sure lots of you can relate to them, though I can't stress enough the difficulty of trying to date when you have the Grim Reaper peering over your shoulder, ready to pounce whenever you believe you're happy or content.

Anyways, getting back to how I met my first serious partner, Louise. Let's face it, that's what you all want to read about. The nitty-gritty. We initially started talking through a chat room. Our relationship grew from there, chatting to each other every day. Roughly six months after we started chatting, we eventually both plucked up the courage to meet.

I was still living in Wrexham. She was one hundred and fifty miles away in Cambridge. We arranged for me to go down to her parents for the weekend. Talking on the telephone and through a keyboard is a vastly different experience to face to face. My nerves got the better off me at first, I spent most of the time talking to her mum and family. I did not know how to talk to her. It's kind of funny to think about it now, but I can recall Louise texting me while we were still in the same room as her Mum. She asked if I liked what I saw and if I was comfortable. She said we could head up to her room for some privacy. My heart started pounding, I had never been alone with a female other than my Mum or sister, oh and the tens of nurses that have attended to me over the years, but this was different. I can remember asking her Mum's permission to go upstairs. Manners and being polite are a top priority for me in life.

Once upstairs in her room, I felt awkward and nervous, unaccustomed to the etiquette of courtship and relationships. I tried to be brave and hide my nerves, but she saw straight through it. She sat on her bed, her back supported on the wall.

She kicked off her shoes and gestured by tapping the duvet for me to join her on the bed. I put my rucksack down on the floor beside her dressing table. Her room was light and inviting, not cluttered but with lots of pictures on the walls.

The window was slightly ajar, and her door firmly closed. "I won't bite you, if you don't want me to!" Louise said with a mischievous grin. I shot her a wide-eyed look and replied, "Steady on, I have not even been here two minutes and you're talking about biting me!" We both fell about giggling like naughty teenagers hiding behind the bike sheds at school, getting up to no good.

I kicked off my trainers and removed my jacket, hooking it over the back of a plush blue suede chair pushed underneath her sturdy pine dressing table, the surface of which was filled with lotions and potions. None of which she needed. She had a smooth complexion that glowed. Her eyes were green and sparkled with kindness. She was heart-warmingly caring and had a deep affection towards me. Her hair fell in glossy lengths just past her shoulders, hair the colour of a golden cornfield with strands of light brown dancing between the rays. Her curvy figure stretched over a slightly taller stature than me: she was five feet six inches of pure gold. (I know what you're thinking, anyone over the age of 12 years would be taller than me, but a wise person once said to me that small things are far more valuable, like the tiny gemstones in the earth. Don't judge something by its size but by its worth, if you should judge it at all).

Her voice was calm and understanding, steady and unrushed. When I was with Louise all my negativity poured from my veins and disappeared from my body. At last, I felt like my life was worth all the fighting and battles won to stay alive.

Her family was very accepting of me and welcomed me with open arms. They took the time to ask me about my life and were in awe of my story. Her mum would make sure I was comfortable and was always offering me food. She made a good brew too, especially after the long tiresome journey on the train down to Cambridge. I think her Mum saw that I was not messing her daughter about and that I was genuinely interested in making a go of things. I so wanted to build a life worth living. My partner would get so sad, when I had to leave, as did I, though she also knew the importance of my treatment. We were getting on so well and our relationship was moving from strength to strength.

I used to try and arrange to travel down to Cambridge every couple of months if possible. This was all dependent on my dialysis access and health condition. Sometimes I was just too weak to travel. We utilised other forms of communication, such as the telephone and the internet. We would talk nonstop for hours. Finally, I felt accepted and had a purpose in my life. It felt like a completely different world when I stayed there, yet most of the time it was only for the weekend.

We made every minute count. Restaurants, cinema, walks hand in hand through the park. My heart couldn't have loved this girl any more, even if I tried.

It felt right and good. I couldn't imagine ever wanting to be with anyone else, or even worse, without my baby girl. I had a brief chat with her mother about our future. I know this was my first girlfriend and I know we were both incredibly young, but it felt extremely comfortable and mutually good between us.

I decided to propose to Louise on her eighteenth birthday. It wasn't the most romantic of proposals, and it wasn't a big gesture or the perfect way I had planned. Back then, I had to do the things that felt right and not stick to the easy things.

Being twenty-one, and with all the things I had gone through, time was precious to me. Being with my partner made me feel valued, loved, and cared for but mostly her affection towards me and her understanding shone from her every pore. I couldn't have been happier. She dedicated her life to me and did everything in her power to make things work between us.

Cracks started to appear. We would often talk about our hopes and wishes for the future and try and make plans, but there was always one subject that would be like the big elephant hidden in the room. We both knew it was there, though we would avoid mentioning it in case we heard something we couldn't accept. One of the hardest things in our relationship was that she had always expressed her need to become a mother herself. At the same time, I was unsure of my fertility due to all my medical issues. We had an active sex life and we meandered fantastically around my dialysis access. She was so gentle and kind, but this led to her feeling like she was the one with fertility issues.

Louise felt as if she had let me down in our quest to become parents and have our own family. She would make comments about her useless body, or she would doubt if she was good enough for me anymore. She would ask me questions, like did I still find her attractive? Did I fancy her? Was she enough? All of the answers were "Yes! Yes! Yes!" But I felt her drifting away from me a little more each day.

I felt anger building inside myself. My body was the issue. It was my fault that we were unlikely to become parents. I felt frustrated that at this point all the medical staff were interested in was keeping me alive. They would talk access points and transplants all day long, yet they would not even consider me for fertility testing. It was not a priority for them, but it was very much so for us. I understood that now was not the right time to start trying for a family, but just having the answers could help heal some of the hurtful wounds being caused by the unknown in our relationship.

I spent a huge amount of time in the hospital and Louise would be sitting at home alone. My health was deteriorating daily, leaving us not knowing what the future held for us. Her need for family was becoming an obsession. The wedge between us grew bigger. After months of self-doubt and some heated arguments, our relationship reached a bitter end.

The hurt was deep and lasting. Even at that moment, I knew this would affect me for many years to come. I let her down and my body failed me.

This was something else I had lost due to my fucked-up body. Now I have a fucked-up mind and spiralling mental health issues to go with my physical health. It's times like this that I feel helpless and wonder what's the point of fighting on. Why should I keep trying a new procedure? I'm not meant to be here, otherwise why would my life need so much of a fight to stay alive? Is it time to cut my losses and say no to any more interventions or dialysis? I had given it a good go. I tried my best. Life sometimes just doesn't work out, and at the moment I couldn't see a reason to fight on.

Unfortunately, after 5 years of an amazing, tiring, straining relationship, we called it a day. We just weren't compatible anymore. It saddens me to admit that even now the pain is at times too much to bear. It's true what people say. Your first love is the one that stays with you for a lifetime. The breakup was tough on us both, my partner moved back home to Cambridge to be supported by her friends and family, which I respected.

How could I not? Afterall Louise was only young when she moved so far away from her family and the familiarity of home. To be with the man she loved is hard in any circumstances, but she did it with the added complexities of the circumstances I was in. She knew I would be on dialysis three times a week.

My limitations meant that we would be unable to live a normal newly defined relationship. I could never truly put into words how grateful I was. She dedicated her time and efforts to me for the five amazing years that we spent together. Even though those years weren't perfect, I still treasured every moment.

I was constantly in and out of hospital, at one point every single month up until I had finally had my 4th and final transplant. That isn't a life for any partner. I felt guilty about the times I was in hospital. I felt like I deprived her of a meaningful relationship and I always felt that she thought she was more like my carer than my life partner. I truly adored her and loved her wholeheartedly. If you love someone so much, the kindest thing to do is to set them free and let them go.

The following months, and even years, were soul-destroying for me. I had had a real shot of happiness and the fairy-tale of living happily ever after. This dreaded debilitating chronic illness stole my future and drove a wedge between me and the girl I so deeply loved and cherished. I still think about Louise frequently and think about what it would have been like if I had gone to live in Cambridge with her. Would things have turned out differently? Who knows what may or may not have happened? The day my relationship ended and I allowed her to walk away was the very same day I made the biggest mistake of my life.

I put my family, especially Kevin, before my partner, which I regret immensely. Some mistakes you never get over. That decision is typical of dumbass me, putting everyone else's happiness before my own. I was forever putting family and friends first. I, of course, was no angel, and this wasn't the main reason we split.

Our relationship was like a constant battle from the start. Having parents who don't like your partner doesn't help in the slightest, always putting the pressure on, and she felt the animosity between my parents and me. In the end, it was just the straw that broke the camel's back so to speak. My heart was broken, and the shards of a broken heart are still as painful as the day it happened, the hurt felt as vivid and clear as the rainbow in the sky.

A note to Louise, the lovely lady that I will forever love and be thankful to have had the pleasure of sharing my life with, even if for a short while. I am eternally grateful for all the love, support, and commitment you showed me during our relationship. I am glad you are happy and have a beautiful family now, though I will forever be saddened and jealous that we were unable to fulfil our dreams together and create our own family as planned. I can only apologise for the hurt you suffered along the way too. Take care and keep smiling your beautiful smile.

Love, Chris.

CHAPTER 15
Fits and Parathyroid

My first episode of a seizure must have been when I was roughly seventeen or eighteen years old, just after I emigrated to Wrexham. I was sitting at the computer typing something up, after which the next bit I remember is my Mum's account of the situation. She says that I shouted to her that I couldn't find a letter on the keyboard. Mum laughed: "What do you mean, it's right there!" She pointed to it on the keyboard with her chunky finger finished with perfectly manicured nails. The next minute I was starting to have a seizure. Mum clambered onto my stiff body, which was jerking and thrashing out. Laying me on the floor away from everything that could become a danger to me, she rang for an ambulance. She then proceeded to call Paul, who luckily was working in the village on his round as a binman. Paul ran along the streets and up the avenue past the house that always over-indulges in Christmas lights or Halloween decorations. They say it's for the children yet there are only a handful of children in the avenue.

Anyway, I digress. Paul was running towards our home when he passed Claire who was waiting for the school bus with her friends. This at once makes Claire suspicious and she shouts after Paul: "What is wrong?" Paul shouts a breathy reply: "Something is wrong with Chris, you go to school and Mum will call the school if it's anything serious". Claire being

Claire, with her 'I do what I want when I want' attitude (which I have always admired) ignores Paul and follows him. Her friends hear the ear-piercing sound of sirens as the blood-curdling sight of the ambulance rounds the corner, screeching to a halt right outside our home. Her friends cling to the arm of Claire's jacket holding her back. Luckily, the school bus followed the ambulance and pulled into the bus stop. Her friends persuaded Claire to get on board and wait for Mum to call the school.

Mum explained later to me that I had a few more mini-episodes while I was in the ambulance. I was rushed straight to the Resuscitation Unit. Mum was told to prepare for the worst. This was due to me not being able to breath independently. I was placed in an induced coma. I also had to endure numerous scans of my brain. (I know right They must have found a brain to be able to scan it. From what I was told, my brain was in my head and not in my feet as the nurses had always joked about). The scans showed I had experienced a mini-stroke, sometimes referred to as a T.I.A (Transient Ischemic Attack) which in some cases can cause seizures. The hospital kept a close eye on me while I was in intensive care.

Mum said I was in a coma for four or five days. Every time I woke, I didn't know who I was, nor did I recognise anyone else. I can't even begin to imagine the kind of anguish Mum and the rest of the family must have been going through at this time. When I asked Mum to tell me about this episode of my life, she found it quite difficult even to tell me the details. She said it was one of the times she truly thought I was not going to pull through and that she was going to have to plan my funeral.

Luckily though I found the strength to pull through yet again. The medical team grew increasingly concerned, especially with the deterioration of my memory. About five or six days in my Aunt Julie came to visit me. I vaguely remember waking up and thinking, I know that voice? When I said her name the family and medical team were so relieved. They monitored my progress closely. I was always being studied by nurses, doctors, medical staff and students. As the days passed, I grew stronger and more alert. My old self was returning. I started to wind up the nurses and be my cheeky self. I could see the family start to relax, their worried frowns were now easing and their smiles would radiate the room. The sound of laughing and chatter could be heard in my hospital cubicle. The doctor came to do his round and he said that I had made great progress, so discharge from hospital was their next goal. I think there was a sigh of relief in unison. Mum shed a lonesome tear, though she said it was tired tears. Her whole demeanour showed it was a mixture of relief and tiredness, fuelled by anxiety and fear. For a Mum to watch her brave baby boy grow to eighteen years old was always going to be an amazing feat. However, after all the medical procedures and interventions to suddenly have all the triumphs stolen so quickly from her grasp must have been a real shock to her. A painful reality check as to how quickly things can change.

Eventually I was released back into the wild. Sorry I mean home. Sometimes it felt like the wild when Claire and I started arguing, as siblings do, and the fights over the TV remote, or what we wanted for tea. God help whoever scoffed the last biscuit or packet of crisps. I think the worst thing was that if Claire left an empty bottle of milk on the sideboard, I would get the blame. There was no consideration for others: if Claire was happy then the rest of us could live in peace, at least until the next argument arose. Family life was bumbling on as normal, or as ordinarily as you can expect when you're dealing with the after-effects of chronic kidney failure and transplants.

Then one day I was finally left alone at home. Now that Mum felt I was over the worst, she finally felt confident enough to leave me alone. That is when the onset of the second bloody episode happened: yet another seizure. Usually if Mum went away, Claire would come to stay with me or Jason. This particular evening was Mum's 40th birthday weekend and Paul had taken Mum away to celebrate. Jason was working away, and Claire was at a friend's enjoying a sleepover. I told Mum I would be fine. I finally convinced her to allow me to stay alone. All I could think about was watching the TV programmes that I chose and that I could listen to my music at the level I pleased.

I had also planned a long soak in the bath without the added interruption of someone needing the loo. You know that chorus of "I need a wee, I'm desperate, how long are you going to be?" This was always after I had traipsed around the whole house asking everyone if they needed the bathroom. I dip my toe in the soothing water to soak away the drama and exhaustion of the day only to have the door hammered moments later as if it was the police gaining entry of a drug den. I'm sure you can all sympathise with this situation, or at least think twice next time you do this.

My aunt and uncle lived next door, plus Gran lived across the street. All I can remember from that night was talking to my partner on the phone. I remember telling her I was experiencing a headache from hell and that I was going to take some painkillers and get myself an early night. I was told later that I had packed a bag, leaving it at the bottom of stairs and I had called an ambulance, knocked next door and then on my Gran's door before coming back and sitting at the bottom of the stairs waiting for the ambulance. When the ambulance arrived, my uncle came running out asking who they were looking for. When they said my name, he told them I was next door. As they looked through the front door, I was having a seizure. I must have known something was very wrong, but I had thought to pack a bag and knock Gran's door. I don't have any recollection of anything after the phone call to my then partner.

The paramedics asked if this had happened before. My Uncle explained it had happened once before, but he didn't know all of my medical history.

He also explained that my Mum was away for the weekend, but Aunty was on the phone updating them on the events as they were happening. My Uncle came in the ambulance with me to the hospital. It was recorded that I had a further two seizures. My Uncle explained later that he was terrified. Mum and Paul came straight back from where they were staying. Mum must have been terrified, along with the guilt of leaving me. But she shouldn't have felt guilt. Her life should not have been put on hold for me, she deserved to be happy and enjoy a night away, especially for her fortieth birthday. The journey to the hospital as described by Mum was "dreadful".

After lots more scans and investigations it was decided that I was needed to undergo another operation. This was to remove my Parathyroid from my neck. These are two little pea-size lumps in your neck. The operation proceeded as smoothly as expected. I was beginning to recover slowly but steadily. But a short while after the nurse had checked on me, I began to feel strange. I had developed breathing difficulties. I pulled the cord and after a short while, a nurse came to check on me. She assured me, after taking my observations, that everything was fine. She then suggested that I was a little anxious and tired and I should try and get some sleep. I did try. It felt like hours later, though in reality only an hour had passed when I began to struggle to catch my breath. I felt like the room was beginning to spin and my blood was pumping ferociously through my veins. My head felt like it was going to combust.

The patient from across the ward became concerned by my movements, and then he became more concerned by my colouration. He said I was purple and making a weird wheezing noise. He pressed the crash call button and nurses and doctors came running from everywhere towards this gentleman. He shouts out to the staff: "Not me! It's the young lad opposite, save him please Lord, save him he is going to die!"

Given the desperation in the guy's voice I knew I was in trouble, but what happened next was more like a murder scene from a scary movie.

Next thing the doctor suddenly takes out his scalpel and slits open my throat. I felt the warm blood running down my neck and all over my top. The doctor jumped on top of me, straddling my limp body and holding pressure as they rushed me back to the theatre. When I woke up, I had wires and tubes everywhere, followed by a young lady's voice saying: "Good morning, honey, don't move, don't worry about all these wires and things. Oh, and Happy Birthday! Of all places to be!" Being confused, I asked where I was. The nurse explained that I had developed a serious blood clot around my windpipe which had caused my breathing difficulties. The crash team had had to release the pressure by creating an incision near my windpipe to help me breathe, then they took me straight to the theatre to sort the clot. The polite me as always just absorbed the information and muttered a quiet, "thank you".

The nurse checks all my drains and machines as the shocking events that sink in. I felt numb with shock, though a strange sense of serenity washes over me. Yet again a brush with death and yet again I outrun the Grim Reaper. The nurse asks me if I would like a drink and advises me that I have some visitors waiting in the family room eager to see me if I felt up to it. I said yes and asked what ward I was on as I didn't recognise the surroundings.

She replied with empathy that I was in Intensive Care. She further explained about the drain in my neck that was to collect any excess blood, plus intravenous antibiotics to prevent infections.

The nurse left for a short moment as I lay, still soaking in the smell and sounds of the room, like the ticking of the white clock that stood to attention on the pale blue wall. The machine's bleeping as it takes readings from my body. The dripping of my blood into the drain attached to the bed tucked out of sight. The remnants of the earlier events still echo in the air. In a split second, the door bursts open, and the familiar faces of Claire, Mum and Paul hesitate as they enter the room. They assess the situation as they scan the room and the bed that my body occupies. Claire goes: "Bloody hell! All this attention for your birthday! Typical, nothing is ever simple with you!" She then starts laughing.

Mum takes my hand and squeezes it so tightly: "Routine operation they said. Nothing is ever routine when you're bloody involved!" I smiled as Paul sat in the chair across from the bed. He just looked at me with a vacant expression on his face. Even he looked dumbstruck this time.

CHAPTER 16

Dialysis Complications

From as far back as 2002 I have had problems with dialysis access in one way or another. There were blood flow issues, infections and there were the complications of blood clots. These are just a few of the problems I endured. Some of these accounts are from the discharge notes I was given when I went home.

Admitted 2/3/2007
Discharged 3/3/2007
Primary diagnosis: collapsed

This 21-year-old gentleman was admitted following a collapse on the renal unit while he was there for Haemodialysis. When his line was flushed, he suddenly felt unwell and his breathing became laboured. The crash team attended; the nurses were concerned his face was swelling. He was found to have laboured breathing, but his chest was clear with no wheeze, his stats dropped as did his blood pressure. He was given iv hydrocortisone considering his clear facial swelling and initially began on iv fluid, although his blood pressure responded relatively quickly. He was transferred to accident and emergency then Overton Ward overnight, where his condition improved quickly. He was observed overnight but seemed fully recovered by the next morning. We arranged for him to have dialysis that day. It is unclear whether this was a vasovagal episode, or an incorrect vial was used to flush.

As you can see this is unbelievably detailed and, typical me, always causing a fuss of some sort. Nothing is ever straight forward or easy.

Admitted 8/1/2007
Discharged 18/1/2007
Diagnosis septicaemia and herpes simplex
Secondary line sepsis

Admitted from the renal unit as a blue light transfer complaining of rigour and high temperature on Haemodialysis, low blood pressure and tachycardia. Blood cultures taken treated with iv vancomycin and gentamicin for a presumed permcath line infection. Symptoms settled gradually but before discharge Christopher developed a pustular rash on the abdominal area, right arm, hand and back. Revealed by consultant dermatologist who diagnosed rash as disseminated herpes simplex. Treated with oral Acyclovir with no progression of the disease. Discharged home with follow up on Haemodialysis once vesicles have dried up.

Line inserted 3/12/2004 removed same day
Newline 7/12/2004
Formation of right fistula 30/8/2005 failed
Formation of left fistula 23/06/2005 failed
Numerous Angiograms
Numerous vascular scans on arms legs chest

The vascular surgeons decided to put a fistula in the top of my right leg, in between my groin and knee. I wasn't overly keen on this idea since the nurses would have to jab needles into that area at least three times a week. I had to quickly get over the embarrassment of that as I accepted this was the only possibility to give me dialysis access. At least until a potential match was found, it had to be done.

I asked many questions but one of my main concerns was the impact on my partners and my sexual relationships. I was still only young, just starting to be sexually active at nineteen years old. I was also unsure if I could have children at this time, but more worrying to me at the moment was whether I would be able to enjoy one of the few activities that I desperately wanted to hold on to: the intimacy of making love and feeling normal, even if for a short while, sometimes if my partner was lucky a little longer depending on my energy levels. This would be a real loss, especially when considering my premature birth, along with the list of medical procedures around my urethra area since I was born.

The consultant was honest with me. He explained that while I was on dialysis it would be hard to test my testosterone levels and my possibility of fatherhood. He said, "it wouldn't be an ideal time to start a family at the moment anyway, your health is our main concern right now. Let's concentrate on keeping you alive before you think about bringing a family into the world. One step at a time Christopher".

The day of the procedure to create a fistula in my upper leg was just like any other routine surgery I had undergone. Surgery to me is like when others visit the dentist. Some people are scared of the sixth monthly dentist visit, though it's something that just has to be done. That's how I think of operations. They are only carried out if necessary, so I just get on with it. That doesn't mean I'm any less scared of the operation than anyone else, but deep down I know that without the operation I'm more likely to die than if I have it. Kind of strange really, writing that. I don't think at the time of surgery, I give the situation as much deep thought as I have while writing these pages. I have come to realise how incredibly resilient and determined I have become. I just want to live. Not a lavish life but a life worth living. One with happiness and love. Maybe even to be loved or respected, and I would like someone to be able to say, "if he can do it then why can't I?" To give hope and courage to others is priceless.

The operation to create a fistula in my leg went well, with no complications. "It will take a few months before we can begin to put needles into it. Hence why we have kept the line in your chest for the time being", said the surgeon.

The line in my chest wasn't working efficiently enough for a decent blood flow, but it did keep me hanging in there. Small mercies and all that. I was on dialysis two days later, on the ward in a special isolation room. They used this room to prevent infections.

I was in the last hour of dialysis for that day, when, all of a sudden, I had this burning sensation in my right leg. It was agony. The nurse did all my observations as normal. This indicated that my blood pressure was up, but that was normal during dialysis. This is due to your heart having to work extra hard to pull the blood through the vessels. I asked the nurse to check my leg. She removed the sheets from my lower body and quickly noticed it was swelling. Within half an hour the pain made me pass out. Dialysis was immediately stopped. The nurse sent for the doctor to examine my leg. He instantly started to arrange yet another emergency procedure in theatre. It was discovered I had a blood clot on my leg. The surgical team rushed to sort the clot and closed me up. Everything was now supposed to be back on track. Or so we all thought.

I went for dialysis a couple of days later. The dialysis unit was a row of beds or chairs with individuals all having blood pumped from their bodies and flushed through many filters before being replaced within their weak map of veins and arteries. Many of the patients are notably older than me and they always seemed bamboozled that I was there at all. Some would mutter amongst themselves. I used to think to myself: "My kidneys are failing, but my hearing is not. Just bloody ask me!" Instead, they would make up a story to fit the demand for gossip or entertainment. Well, I'm sure it helped them pass the time. While I was on dialysis that day my leg started to bleed, only a little at first, then whoosh, the next thing I knew, there was blood everywhere. At first thought it was my line becoming slightly loose, which in itself is extremely rare. I had never known it to happen previously, but then again anything can happen when it comes to me. I called for help and a nurse came over.

As she approached the look on her face was one that could only be described as horror. She quickly shouted for assistance. I had two members of staff applying pressure to my leg to stop the bleeding. Again I passed out. I knew I had passed out because when I came round I was on my way back to the theatre. This time the surgeon decided to leave the wound open to heal naturally.

This seemed to work for a while, but I knew this was not the end of my worries. I was apprehensively waiting for the next instalment of fun and I was not disappointed.

CHAPTER 17
Race Against Time

About 2 weeks after the removal of the second clot in my leg, Dr Robertson came to see me on the ward. He began to talk to me with a tone of seriousness and urgency in his voice. Dr Robertson was always straight to the point, but there was something quite unsettling about him. His stance next to my bed was steady, though he seemed restless on his feet. He smoothed his wild, grey hair as if to soothe his inner self. There was a sense of panic in his voice.

"Christopher, there is no easy way for me to explain this. Keeping access going for you and preventing it from getting infected is becoming an absolute nightmare for the renal, vascular and surgical teams who are all working tirelessly to keep you going and safe.

I can imagine you are feeling exhausted. We have noticed your frustration and discomfort too. Your body is deteriorating quickly. With this in mind, our only plan is the fourth transplant. We need to try our best to get a match. Your best chance of getting this in the time frame that is of any use to you would be a family member. A live donor is your only option right now. Unfortunately, it's difficult for me to say this," he paused and his restless hands came together in a tight clench, so much so that I could see the knuckles on his fingers turning pale. Visibly in turmoil, he accentuated the gravitas of his words with a huge deep breath. "If we are unsuccessful at finding a donor," another deep breath, "we will be lucky to see Christmas 2009".

I was in complete shock. I knew that I had had a lot of procedures recently and that I had suffered hallucinations and blackouts. Was this just a nightmare? Had I become ill again, did I honestly just hear that? Why is this happening? I took a lingering look around the room. I noticed Dr Robertson talking with Julie the nurse in the doorway. I overheard my name being mentioned.

Julie looked over in my direction. She had a look of horror and pity. Her eyes were sad and her face with its ridges of concern put years on her usual youthful complexion.

Dr Robertson rested his expert hand on her shoulder, giving her a gentle steadying. They both looked over towards me. My mind was racing, searching for words to say and thoughts to think. I raised my arm slightly and Julie nodded and made her way towards me.

"Hello, gorgeous!" Her words escaped her lips before she even reached my bed, her smiley disposition trying to break the tension that was building in the space between us. My heart was aching.

I turned away from her to swallow my tears. The lump in my throat would not be helpful so I banished it from view. Julie said again, "hey gorgeous!" as if she was on autopilot. "Do you have any questions?" Immediately my words rushed like vomit from my lips over-spilling the confinements of my mind. "My twenty-first birthday is coming up next year! My partner is coming to live with me once we get our place, will that even happen now?"

Julie smiled with sympathy purring from the corners of her perfectly formed bright pink lips. Her words were unsteady as she replied, "we will do our best. Let's see how Dr Robertson wants to begin his trials. I will be back soon. Are you comfortable?" She plumps up my pillows and offers me my headphones.

Julie knew me better than I knew myself at this moment. I refused but she insisted. I obliged and rested them on my ears. One of my favourite tunes was playing, delicately relieving the pain from my recent news.

Two hours passed. Whilst listening to the melodies playing in my ears, I begin to unravel the nightmare of my news. Julie came back to check my observations. I removed my headphones and asked if she could call Mum. "Can you ask her to come down, tell her I need her urgently." Julie replied, "I'd best get these sheets changed then, your Mum will kill me if she sees the mess I made while trying to be a nurse." I knew she was trying to lighten the mood, but I felt numb.

I had no reply, no quick sarcastic remark, no quip. I just lay there in silence and stillness. In that space of time, my life didn't feel like fun or calm. I just felt disheartened and deflated. The room felt empty and cold. The explosions of colour on the posters on the wall seemed to drain and become dull.

The walls and ceiling and floor became entwined. The ceiling felt like it was squashing down on me, squeezing the air from my lungs. My heart began to race, the pulsing of my blood surging in the cavity of my ears. I felt panic washing over me as the reality of telling Mum that I was dying hit me like a freight train speeding along the rails. An hour passed and still no sign of Mum. Negative thoughts were seeping into my conscience. Had Julie told Mum the news and Mum just didn't care about me? What if Mum and my partner had already been told and had decided to walk away? What if Mum couldn't deal with the news of potentially losing her brave baby boy? How do I tell my family that my body has failed me again? I would be such a disappointment to them all.

I rolled over in the bed to spot Mum arriving with Paul just as Dr Robertson entered the room to check something on my notes. I chickened out of breaking the devastating news to Mum. I just couldn't bring myself to be the one to break her heart. I asked Dr Robertson to explain to them what he had previously told me.

He briefly gave them an overview and told Mum and Paul there was a meeting arranged for tomorrow afternoon. He told Mum to invite Kevin, my father and the grandparents. The meeting would be to discuss Christopher's future. Mum was listening intently. I could see her heart breaking in slow motion through her eyes.

They were always the window to Mum's soul. I could always instinctively know what she was thinking without a word spoken.

The flush of redness on her skin was growing like wild roses up to her neck and flowing over her face, the signs of anxiety and pain that she was desperately fighting to keep locked away, finding the cracks to flow from, like the cracks of a dam under pressure. Mum's chin began to quiver and her eyes filled with helplessness and tears. Paul thanked Dr Robertson for his time and assured him that he would tell the relatives as soon as possible.

Mum and I had been avoiding eye contact until now. Then both of our heads raised just enough to catch a glimpse of the sadness and sorrow in each other's heart.

I had an overwhelming feeling that I had let her down, that my body was getting weak quickly. The very child she had fought to keep alive was fading away in front of her. Mum held out her hand to me in a way that gave me flashbacks to when I was young and holding her hand in the park as we would walk to feed the ducks or walk along the avenue towards Grandma's for a sneaky cake or sweet treat. The smell of sugar and butter being baked is one that makes your senses dance inside, as is the smell of freshly cut grass in the park and the sound of chicks chirping as they leave the safety of their nest for the first time.

What if I never get to experience these things again? Mum's grip grew tighter. In reply so did mine. A signal to one another that what will be will be, but the battle will be fought together.

The sun suddenly burst through the grey sky and filled my room with the brightness of its glory. Even Paul seemed gobsmacked to have received such news today. He was usually quiet and unassuming, though he was trying harder than ever to fill the silence in the room.

The following day came and everyone who Dr Robertson had requested turned up, both my parents and grandparents, even Paul. Kevin seemed rushed, as if he had somewhere better to be. To be fair hadn't we all. Though I knew I was going nowhere fast.

They all came to see me in my bed. Gran bent her head and planted the softest kiss on my forehead, leaving a smear of her lips lingering on my skin. Her perfume filled the air with musk. Grandad shook my hand far more gently than normal. I had instantly braced myself for impact as Grandad could be like a bull in a china shop. "So," Grandad said, while he found himself a chair to rest on, "what's all the fuss about this time lad?" Grandma shot him a look of contempt.

Mum held my hand as she briefly explained what doctor Robertson had told her and Paul last night. Grandad and Grandma looked shocked the same as Mum did yesterday. Their mouths dropped open and their eyes were searching my face for answers. They both looked around the room and then back at me. My drains were still attached, and my wound still open from the blood clot removal some days ago. "I'm so sorry," Kevin muttered. "What's the plan then?" he asked my Mum.

Luckily Mum was saved by the ward manager as she came to explain that everyone from the medical team was in attendance and ready to start the meeting.

Everyone took a breath in unison. It felt that between them they sucked in all the oxygen in the room because my lungs struggled to catch a breath. My anxiety rose again and all I could do was sit and wait. The family all followed the ward manager in a line, which resembled a nursery school trip. "Everyone grab a buddy and follow them in the line", the nursery teacher would say. Mum was first in the line with Kevin at the back.

Kevin kept checking his watch. I wonder what's more important than finding out your child is possibly going to die before he reaches twenty-four?

I didn't go to the meeting, which I found weird. After all, they were discussing the possibility of the last few years of my life. Or was it a meeting to discuss the end of my life? Were they keeping things from me? The wait was hell.

Time seemed to stand still. This must have been how my parents felt during all my major operations. Over an hour later, everyone came out of the meeting. Paul escorted Mum to get some fresh air and a drink. Grandad Howard needed the nicotine fix of a cigarette. Kevin hadn't returned.

Grandma came and sat with me, giving me another one of those wet kisses. I so needed the reassurance that she was giving me in those moments of affection. She went on to explain that they had a few plans of action for me.

The first plan was to reinstate me on the transplant list once they felt that I was well enough.

The second plan was to get as many of the immediate family members as possible tested to start looking for potential matches.

The third plan was to see a bladder specialist to check if my bladder was working efficiently enough for a transplant and wash it out. Along with the transplants, the other idea was that I may need to have a permanent bag, called a Urostomy, attached to my stomach. Grandma was quick to interject, "but don't be thinking about that just yet". All these options that I never knew existed only twenty-four hours earlier. I was finally able to breathe a sigh of relief. "We haven't given up yet," Grandma said, "neither should you!"

Dr Robertson came back on the ward later that afternoon to explain that they were going to place a permanent dialysis catheter into my groin once it was settled and working efficiently enough after a week of dialysis. I could go home with it. He also explained that this dialysis access was my ultimate lifeline. Under no circumstances without his express permission, even if I am admitted to accident and emergency, does that line get used by anyone other than for dialysis purposes. It must never come out. He had written all this in red block capitals across all my notes. He then says, "I'm also explaining to you as you need to understand how important this line is!" I nod in agreement that I fully understand his demands.

The testing for another transplant began.

Julie, the transplant nurse, made appointments for immediate family only to be tested first. Mum was the first in the queue to be tested as I had expected. Unfortunately, she wasn't a match. This news once again broke her heart. She felt useless and thought she was letting me down. Even though I knew in my heart she would die for me if she had to. Paul was next to be tested. Excitedly he passed the first couple of tests. This was shocking to me and Mum as he was only related through marriage to Mum. I was grateful that he even put himself forward for testing. This showed Mum and me his dedication to our family.

Jason my cousin also came forward for testing. I felt incredibly lucky to have these people care enough about me to come forward. Jason passed the first few tests too. Things were looking far more positive than a few weeks ago. Gran on Mum's side also went for tests, though we were braced for a negative result with her. We already knew she had health issues of her own.

Amazingly Uncle Derek also came forward. I was shocked at that decision because he was very scared of hospitals and hardly visited me in all the time I was in here, not because he didn't care but because he was just so scared. Fortunately, he passed the first test but quickly was seen not to be a viable match. Thanks for trying though Uncle Derek, it meant a lot for him to come forward. Aunty Julie (Jason's Mum) wasn't a match though she tried. Thanks, Aunt Julie.

Family and friends from Manchester were tested, though none of them, unfortunately, matched positively.

Grandma Joan had too many health issues to even go through the testing process and Grandad Howard smoked like a chimney so was refused a test. I didn't hold that against them though. They both did everything they could from the day I was born to make me feel loved and cared for and I knew if they could have helped, they would have. Time was not on their side. All three of us were like ticking timebombs.

Kevin was the only person from his side of the family to be tested. This spoke volumes unheard to many. I knew I was never really part of their family. I was just an inconvenience. In all honesty, I was shocked that Kevin himself got tested. Especially as our relationship was quite fractious. Luckily, he passed the first few tests and was going for further tests a few days later.

So far the following people were potential matches: Kevin (my biological father); Paul (Mum's husband); Jason (my cousin). The tests continue as I get a little stronger in hospital and undergo another operation to have the permanent dialysis catheter fitted into my groin. As Dr Robertson said previously, after a week or so of dialysis I finally got home. I finally got to sleep in my bed, even if just for a short while. Life should be for living I thought. I never know how long I have left. So, I started to make plans.

CHAPTER 18

Preparation for Live Transplant and Urostomy

A few weeks pass and the preparations for my live donor are progressing slowly but steadily. The process needs to be thorough and takes an extremely long time. The tests can be tiring, especially for the family members that came forward for testing. They must pass numerous amounts of tests, including blood tests. These tests will determine their compatibility to become my live donor. They also had to undergo ultrasound scans on their lungs, bladder, heart, and kidneys. These scans provide a good measure of their health, making sure they're well enough to undergo the intensity of surgery. It also allows them the best chances of recovery afterwards.

Being a live donor can take its toll, not just on the recipient but on the provider of the transplant too. The donor must make healthy lifestyle changes and commit to them. Changes such as exercise and diet, even their mental state, are examined during the period of offering to donate. The driving force behind live donation cannot be blackmail or coercive control. Another investigation that is made is to see if there has been a conversation around money regarding the donation. The transplant team must be 100% sure that the reasons for offering to donate are completely ethical and legal.

These are the most common questions donors ask.

- What are the risks of my surgery?
- What will you do to reduce those risks?
- How much pain will I be in?
- What will you give me to relieve pain?
- How might this surgery affect my life afterwards?

(*These questions were sourced from MD*)

My chances of receiving a donation from family seemed to be slipping away. Week by week a different family member would fall at each hurdle. Jason fell first after a scan revealed an anomaly in one of his organs. Jason was devasted and took a real hit for quite a while. He felt helpless and worthless. We had been so close growing up and more like best buddies than cousins. He would protect me at school and was always there to defend my honour. In his eyes, the time I needed him the most he was unable to save my fading life. Jason started to avoid my calls and would make excuses if I invited him round.

The decision of the transplant team has to be final. After all, it's life and death. They wouldn't want Jason to need medical assistance for the rest of his life for the sake of helping me to prolong mine. This would be unethical and not economically viable. The decisions that are made during the process of testing have a substantial effect on the lives of everyone involved. It brings into question the loyalty of those around you. Then there's the effect of the overall decision to consider. The donors may feel worthless, failure or resentment, sometimes even self-shaming that they were unable to help, though there is counselling available for all involved.

After a week or so I reconnected with Jason and with the help of other family members we were able to reassure him that he did not let me down as he thought. In my eyes he was a hero. He stood up and put himself forward yet again to save my ass. Just like he had done in all the other scrapes and I had got myself into over the years, mainly at school or on the playing fields. Jason has proved time and time again that he had my back when others just turned a blind eye. For this I will always be grateful to him.

Another week or so passes and so were my donors. This time it was Paul's turn to be let slip. Mum looked so disappointed when Paul was called into the hospital office by Dr Robertson to be told, "Unfortunately, we feel at this stage it would be unfair to proceed with your tests. You are no longer able to donate to Christopher at this time". He went on to give the usual baloney about heroism and offering counselling. But none of these things prolong the life of the dying or comfort the failure felt by the donor in that instant.

Mum took the news hard and this caused fractures in her relationship with Paul for a short while. The disappointment and sorrow felt by Mum was evident in the slamming of doors, as the harsh reality rushed towards her. The likeliness of losing her son was like a train heading towards her. Her world was unravelling before her eyes. The courage within her to keep positive was fading like the day's light. At sunset that evening the mood at home was fraught with disappointment, anger and sadness. Paul headed to the pub for some much-deserved solace and to be alone with his thoughts.

For Paul, not only had he let down his stepson, but he had also failed to honour the love and steadfast loyalty for his wife, my mother. I could feel the tension rising and felt responsible. I was in despair to think that the rift in the home was caused, yet again, by my failing, deteriorating body. My own mental state was not much better if I was honest. I respected Paul for even offering to be tested let alone going as far as he had. This to me showed more spirit and loyalty than ever. He did not have to go through the relentless tests and scans, but he did. He knew what it meant to Mum, especially after her earlier disappointment of falling at the first test.

This left me with Kevin as the only option. So far, he was still in the running to be the one to make a difference. Though this put questions in my head I did not voice them or even let on to anyone. Afterall, I want to live and if I was to even suggest hesitation in the idea that Kevin was now, fingers crossed, to be my lifeline then that option would also be dismissed. No, for the sake of life I would swallow all my pride and smile gracefully that Kevin was still in the mix for lifesaving transplant surgery.

The next few days were crucial. I attended the dialysis unit and had all my lines checked. I felt nervous when I arrived at the unit. I'm not sure why, but there was an overriding feeling of apprehension and anxiety. I felt butterflies in the pit of my tummy and the instant I clapped eyes on Julie, the transplant nurse, in a meeting with Dr Robertson I knew my fate was being discussed. I could just tell. Sally, the dialysis nurse, greeted me at the reception area of the unit. Her sparkling smile was glowing brighter than I had noticed before. Then Helen, a young student nurse training on the unit, came to show me to my throne for the next eight hours of dialysis. "Get yourself comfortable," she said in her hushed tones. Her nerves were visible on her first day. Her hands were shaking while holding my notes. "I will be back to weigh you and take your blood pressure in a minute. I just need to ask where the machine is?"

Her honesty was her best feature, it was quite endearing. But I was feeling more exhausted than ever. When the young nurse said I had to wait, a wave of frustration and anger rose in my throat. I couldn't be bothered to be messed around or having to wait. I just wanted to be hooked up and feel better, as quickly as possible. I rolled my eyes at the young nurse and hissed a sarcastic remark, which obviously hit a nerve with her. She stormed off and within a moment Sally's cheerful disposition filled the area. "Stop being a diva!" she shot at me. "You're not royalty yet, so don't start acting like one. Helen has been here less than an hour and she has had the raff off you. Play nicely!" Helen returned with the machine to take my temperature and blood pressure and quickly wheeled in the scales to check my weight too. I could see the slight run in her mascara from tears she had shed after my scolding.

"I'm sorry," I muttered sheepishly. "I'm just struggling with all this and feel so tired. It's no excuse to take the frustration out on you though." Helen smiled and said, "no problem, it's just part of the job description: emotional hitting stick, here for all to shout at and demand things from". She recorded my numbers in my notes and awaited the next instructions from Sally. Helen then made idle chitchat by saying, "Dr Robertson wants to see your notes before we can proceed today. He is going to give you some news on your live donor depending on these results. He is waiting for Kevin to arrive." While I sat there mulling over what Helen had said I saw my father come into view through the glazed wall of the dialysis unit. My heart felt like it had stopped. My breath caught in my lungs. My fate was to be decided on my numbers and on the results of Kevin's tests.

Just then I saw Mum enter the reception area too. She and Kevin share a pensive nod and are shortly joined by Paul. What the hell is going on now? Why are they all here? What am I not being told this time? Everyone seemed melancholy and glum. All except Sally of course, her cheerful humming serenaded the whole unit while her perfume disguised the clinical smell of sterile equipment. Her calming way soothed the most painful days. With that Dr Robertson's door swung open with force. His tall outline came into view along with his gingham red shirt and beige chinos, and his giant size tan leather shoes freshly polished the previous evening. He treads the tiled floor towards my bed, with my files tucked neatly under his left arm. He pauses only to collect the soap at the hand-wash basin. He washes his hands and takes two paper towels to dry them. He throws away the dampened paper towel and makes his way to me.

His big brown eyes catch sight of my dark-circled tired eyes. He asks me how I'm feeling, then begins to talk. "Listen up," he says. "We are in a real dilemma here. Your body is weak and your fight to survive can only be described as dwindling. If we are going to have any chances of a viable transplant, I think we should start the last stages. Kevin is your only hope and luckily for you all the tests suggest that we are on the right track. There are a few more boxes that need ticking but I'm staying focused and so should you." I felt my body relax and the breath caught in my lungs finally found a way out. Hopefully my fortunes were changing. I lay back on the slightly reclined chair while Sally attached all my lines, starting my dialysis.

Dr Robertson nods to bid me farewell and says, "Now to break the news to the family. Not long now, Chris, and we will do our utmost to make you feel a little more comfortable." With that he made his way back to his office, my notes still tucked under his arm. As he approached my family in the reception area, they all stood to attention like soldiers in the forces. I could see Dr Robertson's face from my position, and I could see his amusement though I could not hear the conversation. The family followed him into his office.

I must have dozed off. When I woke, my curtains were closed around me and my immediate area was full. My family and

Dr Robertson all had a more optimistic sense about them. All except for Kevin. Kevin looked scared out of his wits. "Right then Christopher, we have a plan!" said Dr Robertson. "I will go make some calls and then be back. Kevin can break the news to you and fill in the gaps. I will be back in a short while if anyone has any questions." Off he went back to his lair, or office as some know it.

Kevin stood there in utter silence, alone in his thoughts. I understood that in a way. I noticed the colour draining from his face. "You best get him a seat," I said to Mum, "he doesn't look too well". Mum laughed and said, "he will be ok, he has just been told that he is going to be the chosen one. The hero of the day. Kevin has passed all tests to become your live donor. Dr Robertson wants to get everything in order in the next few months or so. There is still the matter of your bladder that needs addressing before the transplant can happen." Kevin lifted his head momentarily and smiled straight at me. He then whispered, "if you still want to go ahead with the transplant that is?"

"If not, I die," I shot straight back. "I have no choice really, do I?" Mum explained that Kevin and I had to go to see a psychiatrist. I think this was to make sure no one was being pressured into being a donor or that the donor wasn't getting paid to donate. It felt like a crazy process we had to undergo, though I understood the necessity of it in some cases.

A few months passed and it was now mid-June. I booked into the Manchester Royal Infirmary to have a procedure done called a Urostomy. This was a procedure to make a stoma into my stomach in order for me to pass urine. This the consultants felt would be my best option in order to reduce the risk of UTI's and water infections. This meant that I had to have a permanent bag attached to me. It was not the best idea for me but the one I had to go with. The operation itself was not too difficult or scary. What was scary was the impact it may have on my life, my sex life, my relationships and my social life. My mind was again racing with all the things good and bad about this procedure. At the age of twenty-one, I'm more like an incontinent geriatric than a young man in his prime.

The Urostomy bag also meant that I would always be carrying a bag of piss around with me. The hygiene routine alone of this was yet another thing for me to have to learn, along with how to overcome my embarrassment and awkwardness when it came to getting frisky with the missus. What impact is this going to have on her? Would it get in the way of sexy time? I have spoken to doctors and they say we will work it out, but I'm not sure. The consultant and transplant surgeon felt that if my body could cope with this operation, I was all clear to go ahead with the transplant. Having a Urostomy was a completely new thing to get used to. It was just there not doing anything until I had the transplant. I wasn't passing any urine through it so it had no purpose as yet. It was just an ugly and useless add-on. A reminder that me and my body were damaged goods for all to see.

Thankfully the operation went well considering the strain my body was going through. Now I just had a few weeks to recover and for Kevin to organise his time off work and his other commitments, affording him the time to donate his kidney to me and to give himself sufficient recovery time. Kevin was not good at sitting around and being lazy but this time it was essential that he just takes the time to allow his body to heal. Kevin visited me a few times while I underwent the boring process of dialysis. I think it was more for his benefit than mine. I think he treated it like a practice session of sitting still for prolonged periods. I think Kevin gets the raw end of this donor malarkey, of which I will always be grateful. If I'm entirely honest though, I do feel a real sense of expectation with him giving me his kidney.

I feel the pressure to make this work and last for as long as possible. If it was to fail, then I would be letting Kevin down. He is giving up his kidney to save the life of his son, yet, if it was to fail it will let him down and waste his body parts. The emotional labour these decisions cause and the family dynamics are already complicated. Then to add the gift of live donation from a family member, and being a recipient has always filled me with trepidation and worry. But without Kevin gifting me this lifeline, the reality is that I will DIE.

The last time I had haemodialysis at Wrexham dialysis unit was an emotional experience. This had become my life for the last seven years. The nursing staff were now my extended family.

I knew them all on first name terms. I always did my best to make them laugh or help them with the latest technological devices. I even gave recommendations of gifts for loved ones, especially around Christmas time. Sometimes I would be sitting at my laptop checking stock levels for their Christmas list while they were working. I know this was all part of them making me feel comfortable and settled, the art of misdirection and distraction that all nurses are taught in med school. The practice worked. I did truly feel like I was just one of the team. Some days I would even forget why I was there. It felt like visiting family or friends. I always have a sense that I owe those nurses my life. They always did their best to make my life as simple and positive as possible. I felt they all went above and beyond the call of duty for me. They made me feel special in my time of desperation.

The next step would be the transplant. The tensions were rising in both Kevin and me. I became quite emotional, in private of course. Men in my family were never allowed to show emotion, especially sadness or fear. No crying allowed. We are a military family with a British stiff upper-lip. No tears fall on these cheeks. I received a call from Kevin that evening. He talked nonsense mostly, but he did show his vulnerability and the fear could be heard in his voice, double-checking the details and going over and over the arrangements and times for our procedure. In the end I was the one to say goodbye. I told him to go make sure he got some sleep and took a long soak in the bath. Bathing would be out of the question for a while. Bed baths and strip washes were now going to be his new way of life for the next few weeks, along with hospital food and lazy days. "See you in the morning, Dad", I said. "Oh, in case I have not said it enough times, thank you for trying. No matter what the outcome, thank you for trying." "See you tomorrow, Chris," Dad replied. I turned off my phone and lay down, music in my ears and before I knew it I had drifted off.

CHAPTER 19

Kidney Transplant from Kevin

29th October 2009. This date is hopefully the last time I will ever need to undergo this procedure. Surely there can't be a better match than your own parent's kidney? I was so nervous arriving at the hospital with mum, my partner, Louise, and Paul. I underwent all the usual protocol of the previous procedures. However, this one felt very different. The experience is full of deep emotion and expectation. The trepidation is far worse when I know the donor. I had a lot of anxieties running through my mind. Would I make it through the operation? What if Kevin changed his mind and can't go through with it? What if we go through this ordeal and it fails straight away? What would he think of me if it fails in the future?

The operation is the most nerve-wracking I have ever experienced. I hadn't seen Kevin since the night before. I can only imagine the feelings travelling through his mind, though I'm sure they would be similar to mine at present. I lay upon the bed in the anaesthetic room and it felt like I was there for an eternity. I could hear people talking. My mind playing the paranoid trick that it regularly plays when relying on others. I always await the disappointment of being let down. My thoughts start racing. The thought of Kevin getting all the way to anaesthetics and changing his mind. Maybe the realisation and fear have overwhelmed his thoughts. What happens now?

The next thing I see is the nurse making her way towards me, looking at me with a comforting smile. She tells the staff, "we are ready", and with one sweeping move the mask is placed over my face, covering my mouth and nose while they reminded me to stay calm and to slowly start counting backwards. In an instant I start counting sheep and dreaming. The procedure begins. Time passes and finally the procedure comes to an end.

After a while I open my eyes surrounded by machines yet again playing their own rhythmic melody of bleeps. The recovery trolley feels uncomfortable under my weak body. The buzz of the staff around me feels different to before. There seems to be an excitement fizzing in the air. As I move my head to glance around the room a figure catches my eye. It was Kevin. He was on a trolley over towards the far end of the room. He raised his hands above his head and gave me a little wave. There were no words shared between us, but it was a signal for us to communicate the success of transplant. Now the agonising wait begins, to see how successfully my fourth transplant turns out.

As the nurse checked over me and recorded my observations, she asked her normal mundane questions. How are you feeling? How do you think I'm feeling, I thought to myself. I have just had my insides messed with and now you're asking how I feel? How do you think the clothes feel when tossed and tumbled in a washing machine? Being my usual polite self, I just nodded and said yes. The nurse then proceeded to explain that I had also been fitted with a Urostomy.

This Urostomy was a weird thing to get used to. Especially the process of cleaning and adhering to the hygiene rituals. Then there is the cutting of the bag to make sure it's securely stuck to me in order to last a maximum 48 hours to prevent infections. Not only had I undergone another procedure,

I now needed to learn a new way of going to the toilet and dealing with the complications and embarrassment of sporting a Urostomy bag.

There are complications that those of you who are lucky enough not to need one would overlook. Things like how the bag needs to be held securely. What happens when my bag leaks? This is like regressing back to my childhood and peeing the bed, only this time I'm grown up and it's not my fault. Nevertheless, this is still embarrassing when sharing the bed with my partner. However, keeping perspective, I was alive and hopefully I would be able to live my life to the best of my ability.

Recovery went as smoothly as it could for me, and after a few weeks in hospital I returned home. Kevin also recovered well. For now, life had been re-started, but this is me and my body: it won't last forever.

CHAPTER 20

Grandad

I am the strong, resilient and courteous person I am today, regardless of all my pain and discomfort, thanks mostly to my Grandad. He was the most influential person in my life. He truly made me the man I am today. He taught me so many life lessons, such as:

To gain respect you must first and foremost earn it.

Always smile because a smile will brighten anyone's day.

Always be polite, well-mannered and make eye contact when talking, it shows you are paying attention and are showing respect.

Howard, my Grandad, was born 4th March 1939. He was a butcher in his teens working in his father's shop. Grandad used to tell me of how he met Grandma (Joan) while he was working in the butcher's shop. I can never recall which way round it was, but they met either while doing deliveries to the same house or when he was delivering meat to the bakery my grandma was working at. They got married when they were 18 and had four children: Linda, Tony, Kevin (my Dad) and Adrian. I have lost count of how many grandchildren and great-grandchildren are in the family.

Howard was in the army for a while but all I remember is him being a local bus driver. He was always there for me. He was the one person I could always rely on. The best way to describe Grandad would be the old man from Disney's "Up" movie. He would always wear his hat and use a walking stick.

When I was around 6-8 years old, he would say he was going to check on the tomatoes in the greenhouse with his dog Charlie and I would say, "Grandad, you've only just been out? Have you got to give them lots of water and attention otherwise they won't grow?" As I got older, I began to realise that he was hiding in there, away from Grandma and having a sneaky cigarette. Other things I fondly remember is when we used to go out for pointless drives together. Grandad's home cooking was the best. I used to get excited when I would spot the Tupperware tubs full of his home cooking hidden in his bag when he visited me in hospital. Grandad would say he was making sure (in his words) I had a proper meal.

Grandad changed his religion to Muslim many years before I was born. I never knew this though until I was in my late teens or even my early 20's. It made sense when I found out as every year he would go on holiday to Pakistan for the whole of February. Sometimes he would miss my birthday, though more surprising he would always miss Grandma's birthday and Valentine's Day. Nevertheless, typical Grandad, he would always be back for his own birthday.

The last time I ever saw Grandad was when myself and Kevin's partner took him to the airport for his annual holiday. At the time of his holiday, he would always see everyone, give them a hug and say see you when I am home. I recall something strange the last time though. He only gave hugs to the youngest members of the family. I remember saying to Kevin, "that's weird!" My curiosity left me in turmoil for a while as he was always so loving towards us all, especially Grandma. At the airport he didn't even kiss Grandma or give her a hug, which was very unusual

When Grandad checked in at the airport we said, "have a good time, see you soon!" Grandad looked at me and said, "Christopher, I love you and will always be proud of you." He spoke those words directly to me and made eye contact with me. I felt a surge of emotion and a deeper connection than I had ever felt before. I knew Grandad's words were sincere and genuine. Grandad's words reached into my body and penetrated my heart, like a spear. Overwhelmed with emotion, the tears built and I felt unsteady inside. I went to give him a hug, but he wouldn't let me. He made it clear not to touch him. He also refrained from giving Kevin's partner a hug too. We found his demeanour and his reactions extremely strange.

The day I got the dreaded phone call, Mum rang me saying, "get a bag packed because Paul is on his way to collect you." I knew something was amiss. Mum's tone of voice sent shivers through my veins. I felt an impending loss. My whole being felt cold and empty, full of loss, yet I had no idea what it was or who it could be. When Paul arrived, I quizzed him. Unfortunately, he had no more knowledge than me. He said, "honestly I don't know, your Mum just told me to come and get you urgently, she said she will explain more when we are all back together." In the meantime, Mum had made a call to Claire. She demanded that Claire return home at once.

I walked in, with Paul closely following. Claire was sat on the sofa with Mum walking around in anxious circles. Claire asked Mum what was wrong. Having experienced these strange feelings, and always putting my foot in it, I just blurted out: "Who has died?"

I could tell it was going to be bad news. Mum instantly broke into tears and told us after a short pause. She took a breath as she looked up, saying, "it's Grandad!"

Claire and Paul instantly burst into tears. I was in complete shock. My brain could not compute what my ears had just heard. I couldn't believe it. I then began asking questions about how it could have happened. Mum began to explain that Kevin had received a call from Pakistan explaining that Grandad Howard had died peacefully in his sleep. I briefly heard Paul say in slow-motion, "when is the funeral?"

"Tomorrow," Mum replied. Claire was confused, asking Mum, "how can it be tomorrow when he is in Pakistan?" Mum further explained that because Grandad is Muslim, their religion denotes that their followers are to be buried within 24 hours after their passing. Grandad's wish was to be buried over there, so we never got to say goodbye and that has always left me with a feeling of unfinished business, and sadness from missing the chance to give Grandad a send-off fit for a king, as to me he was the king of my life and castle. So, I wrote him this message to help settle my heart.

"Grandad, you were truly my best friend. Gone but never forgotten. Rest in peace. Love Christopher."

But the feeling of emptiness and sadness has never left me since that day. I think of him all the time and wonder what he would make of the world today and how I have continued to battle my illness. I think he would be proud as I always promised to make him proud.

CHAPTER 21

Childcare Course and a Traumatic Relationship

Again, after another glitch, I managed to pick myself up and get back on the ladder of life. My life began to take on a sense of normality, even if it were to turn out to be a momentary reprieve. I chose to follow my dreams and train to become a childcare practitioner. This was a one-year childcare course studying at Yale college in Wrexham. Commencing in September 2012, the course was everything I had hoped for. More importantly, I was doing great with my assignments. As part of the course, I was also having to undertake practical assessments in the form of placements. My first placement was in a primary school. I just loved the enthusiasm of the children, and the staff were also very accommodating and understanding of my ongoing health issues. I felt so accepted and part of the team that I was offered a teaching assistant job by the head teacher. They were very impressed with how I interacted with the children and the other staff members. I was always willing to get stuck in and wanting to learn new things or understand their way of learning. I was so over the moon to be offered a permanent position once qualified. I felt very proud of myself and this helped to build my confidence and self-worth. I may have my down sides, but I can still be part of a growing community and do some good.

Whilst things were positive with my career and training, in my personal life there were cracks beginning to show. I was having some serious issues at home with my relationship. Things came to a head just before Christmas. Allegedly I lost my temper in my college class. My relationship was now affecting my training and career path.

My Tutor asked me to step away from my course and take some time to sort my issues out. I was expected back after a week if I felt ready.

After I had taken the week to sort things at home, I went back to college. I was later called into the course leader's office to be told that I was suspended from the course for anger management reasons. This was absurd. This could go on to ruin any future career prospects or training. What's worse is that I would never be allowed to apply for another childcare course nor work with children again in the area. I was fuming and felt so worthless. A moment of frustration and annoyance had been taken out of context and made to be something it was not. Even my gender was used against me in the meeting, along with my health concerns.

I felt disheartened and useless. Again another rejection. Again another person telling me that I was not good enough, or that my flaws caused concern. My body had been failing me for years and I was used to that and had a strategy for dealing with the disappointment of that. But having another person tell me that I'm not good enough is something I will never get used to and it caused me huge anxieties, sparking my depression. The lack of support from my partner at the time also sent me into a spiral of dark thoughts that flooded my mind. My partner would tell me daily I was not good enough and that she could do better. She would control my every thought, feelings and whereabouts.

When I got to Mum's later that day, I explained to her and Paul what had happened. They both thought this was some kind of joke. Unfortunately, it was not. I still don't know the actual reason why I was suspended. Although I was told to leave, it was never explained why. I have my own ideas, but I can never be sure. Yes, I was a little inquisitive, and I would always question the reasons for doing things, but if that's a sackable offence I will never get work or training. It's just the way I am. I like to find out what, where and why. Maybe this is because of all the medical interventions and having to know about them. I think my tutor and I clashed personalities, and the fact that I was the only male on the course was a real issue for the tutor. There were a few passive-aggressive comments made during the lessons.

Me being me though, I just walked away. I was not willing to fight for something again, with the added difficulty of the problems in my relationship with my partner. I was tired of fighting for everything in life. I took the self-loathing route instead. Maybe this was weak of me, but at the time I just didn't feel strong enough to take on another battle. So my spiralling mental health was kicked again. I often wonder what the point of fighting is. I never seem to be happy or content for long.

Partners take advantage of my insecurities and weakness and I never get back the effort that I put into the relationship. One of the hidden issues when dealing with chronic health conditions and hidden disabilities, is that people feel that you are of less value to others. I feel that when finding partners, they either feel sorry for me and want to mother me, or they want to control me. They take advantage of my struggles and run circles around me. Other issues such as financial abuse and discrimination happen all the time. People forget that I'm human and think that its ok to lie or cheat on me. One of my ex-partners told me I should be appreciative that she even touched me when she did because a lot of people would be repulsed by my scarred, under-developed body. I craved to feel loved and wanted. All I desired was to feel supported and needed. I have always had body image issues, but the emotional abuse inflicted by partners and people I have encountered just increases the feelings of worthlessness.

I always stand by the saying: 'treat others how you would like to be treated'. This is so easy to do but so many forget the virtue of this. The way people treat others with disabilities, whether it is hidden or not, has a lasting effect on the well-being of the sufferer. It can be as damaging as domestic violence. Hopefully one day my life-jigsaw will be complete and I will finally get to fit each piece perfectly to allow me true happiness and contentment.

CHAPTER 22

Grandma

When I was around twenty-eight, I made a massive decision to move back to Manchester due to my deteriorating mental health. The way I was being treated by my ex at the time made the decision to leave Wrexham and move somewhere more familiar to me a necessity. In my mind I thought going back to where I grew up, being closer to Grandma, Kevin, Matthew and Mark would provide me with more support and help to develop a social life. That is what I needed to get back on track.

At first, things weren't too bad, but things always seem better at first. I assume that that's down to the change from the norm.

Getting a new consultant, plus transplant team, was a real eye-opener in a major city compared to a town like Wrexham. The units were as busy as the hustle and bustle in the streets and the nurses were less friendly. They didn't have time to chat and do small talk. In Manchester the nurses treated you more like numbers, and the consultants had time slots and schedules to keep. The quality of treatment was good, and the treatments were efficient, thanks to the extra funding and resources that a larger city and major hospital could offer. It was more the personal touches I missed and had undervalued in Wrexham.

The first place I had, when I finally found a suitable one, was a little one-bedroomed ground floor flat in the same village as Kevin, Grandma and Mark. It was ideal and was even on a major bus route. This allowed me the freedom I had lacked in Wrexham. I missed seeing family and friends more than I had ever realised.

The flat was the old village police station, which had been redeveloped into flats. My flat was the old main reception area, where they booked in the criminals. Underneath the building were the old cells. I was told all this by the lady who lived above me. She was lovely, very friendly. We would always stop for a chat if we saw each other. She never complained about my music, though I was respectful and tried to keep it to a minimum. I have always used music as a coping strategy for stress, pain or loneliness.

Manchester made me feel surrounded by kindness and I always felt at home there. I always felt like I belonged. Things started to change when Grandma become more dependent on others and she would ring me all the time, sometimes to do jobs in her flat or pick up her shopping or medication. At the start I felt needed and important to someone, but this started to get a little overwhelming. I thought it was maybe because she was lonely and wanted some company. It was nice seeing relatives and, at times, old friends who I had grown up around. But Grandma became so demanding that I would be running around for her and neglect my own health.

Unfortunately, I had to move out of the flat when the landlord sold it to the Council to provide accommodation for vulnerable adults. I was devasted. The flat had provided me with stability and my own safe space. The Council insisted I moved out, because in their eyes I wasn't vulnerable enough. So, I had no choice but to move in with Grandma, which wasn't a bad short-term idea. I was there all day most days anyway, doing whatever she demanded, but long-term this was not my life's plan. After all I was single and would be able to help Grandma out a bit more while I lived there.

During my short say with Grandma, she started to have carers come in. I grew increasingly concerned about her mental health. She seemed very forgetful and her hygiene routines were not as they had been. The problems, I faced when asking for assessments on Grandma were that health care professionals and Social Services would do mental capacity tests and Grandma passed these all the time. It became extremely tiring and frustrating, let alone mentally draining for me. It felt like no one believed what I was trying to say, apart from family, who had experienced the difficulties too. The main issue I was finding was trying to get a doctor to come and assess Grandma.

In my opinion, at the time the social care system for the elderly was absolutely appalling. They never listened to a word that family members told them, nor did they listen to their own care workers. I just wish I had heard about, or even studied, the Code of Practice for Care Services back then like I have now. I honestly don't think any of it was being professionally used at that time. The assessors were just taking what Grandma was telling them as the truth without clarifying with those who were involved with her on a daily basis.

The social workers would only ever see myself, and mainly Grandma, for most meetings, do a review, put it in place, then we would never see or hear from them again. Three months later it was back to square one. A new social worker and a new process all over again. This must have happened 4-6 times over the 3 years I was in Manchester.

Falls, ambulances and accidents became more frequent and even that was not a spur to further assessments.

Grandma was starting to have lots of issues with her balance, hygiene, memory and infections. It was getting so bad that I didn't know if she was going to bed fully dressed and

I honestly just had to take her word for it about having a wash. There were numerous issues between myself and Grandma, as well as the doctor and chemist over her diabetes treatment. She would tell me she had ordered medication and when I went to the doctor's or chemist's it hadn't been ordered. This then led to her becoming prone to infections due to poor hygiene and missed medication.

The falls were becoming increasingly frequent and the paramedics were coming two or three times a week. They all became familiar with the address and would know all about Grandma, even the call centre staff would know her. The problem was that when she had a slip or a fall it was due to being dehydrated or to diabetic hypoglycaemia low blood sugar levels. I couldn't physically pick her up due to her size and my own limitations.

Kevin was her next of kin, but he would turn his phone off at night. I was next In line to call but it got to the point where the care call company would automatically call me. This was obviously before I moved in with Grandma. Most of the time these calls were between 2 am and 5 am.

Sometimes I would be up all night waiting on an ambulance and by the time they came to examine Grandma she had come round. That is no disrespect to the amazing work the ambulance service provides. Just the way things were.

I would notify Kevin around 7-8 o'clock the following morning as he was getting ready for work. I can't ever fault the paramedics, but by the time they managed to see Grandma it was as if nothing had happened and she would always refuse to go to the hospital to be checked out. even when I had numerous ambulance call-out sheets.

Grandma's behaviour was shocking and seriously rude at times, with no manners, respect or dignity towards anyone or anything apart from herself. She would call demanding I come round straightaway, the assertiveness in her voice making me concerned that it was serious and most times it would be to make a cup of tea, a meal, or wanting her tv magazine for next week even when it had not been delivered to the shops yet.

The arguments about this specific magazine! OMG! I can't begin to describe the heartbreak, anger and disgust that I felt at the way Grandma would talk to me and treat me. The worst things I can ever recall in the times I was helping her were when I would spend numerous hours cleaning the flat after her accidents, and she would tell me that I had not done it correctly, or not to bother next time because I had made it worse. She would treat me like rubbish after spending hours upon hours in Accident and Emergency with her, having to sit there listening to her lies that there wasn't anything wrong with her apart from her diabetes. She would cast aspersions that I just wanted to get rid of her and imprison her in a care home.

The ultimate worst moment was the time my uncle and I brought Grandma back from the hospital and we unlocked the front door quickly as she was complaining she was desperate to use the bathroom. When she had walked halfway up the hallway with her Zimmer-frame, she suddenly took off her incontinence pad, which she used in case of accidents. What came next filled me with horror. Without any warning, she launched her pad straight at me. I stood there in total shock. The pad hit me straight in the face. To rub salt into the wound, she then shouted at me to clean it up!

"After you have finished doing that," she said, "you can make me a brew and go chippy". These were the times when I felt most despair as a result of her actions. I knew that Grandma didn't intentionally treat me this way, but her actions and behaviour always seemed to be aimed at me. She never gave a thought that I had been at the hospital all night and had not slept or eaten properly. All I had managed to do was keep my fluid intake up to ensure I could take my medication. I felt like a walking zombie. This was the last straw, I felt utterly exhausted, downtrodden and helpless. My tears started to rise, though the anguish rose quicker. My head was spinning and desperation filled my head. I could not take any more. I opened the front door, walked out and, before I knew it, I had left her on her own. I was heartbroken: this was the catalyst to my own nervous breakdown.

Grandma unfortunately began to deteriorate without constant help from myself and the carers. She was in and out of hospital with falls and numerous infections, which in turn exacerbated her mental health and her ability to stay at home was reduced. The family had to make the horrendous decision to have Grandma placed in a residential home. Though the decision was made in regard to her own safety, it didn't make it any easier. This may sound harsh and a little selfish, but it also allowed me to regain my life and some of the independence that I had been working towards for so long.

Regardless of how difficult things were with Grandma and how demeaning she was to me, I know in my heart that, if needed, I would do it all over again for her. Living with Grandma was hell as it was so painful to see someone that I loved drifting away. The person I had grown up around had changed and I watched her hour by hour, day by day, morphing into the stranger that she had become. I remember Grandma saying to me when I moved in with her that I wasn't ever to let anyone sell her home.

However, I know I could not promise as it was out of my control. Her children would be the ones to make that decision. After all, I was just the person who was having to look after her and deal with most of her issues. I was an easy option for Kevin and the rest of the family. It didn't matter to them if I was abused or if I was treated badly. It's just me. They never saw the extent of Grandma's behaviour or her hurtful words.

The day the manager from the care home came over to the house to see Grandma, she explained that there was a temporary space available for the next two weeks that Grandma could try out. This was to see how she would feel about having constant care and all her meals prepared for her. The manager was very kind and understanding about all the mixed feelings surrounding putting loved ones into a care facility.

She also explained to Grandma that it was becoming impossible for carers and myself to look after her.

She pointed out to the rest of the family that even if my health was in a perfectly normal state, caring for Grandma would be extremely difficult, never mind with the restraints of being a kidney transplant patient and other medical conditions. She expressed her amazement that I had coped this well for this long. She explained to the family that Christopher was extremely exhausted, mentally and physically. Grandma looked straight at me, with the lady, the social worker, the carer supervisor, Kevin and my Grandma's eldest granddaughter in the room. Grandma turned to me and begged me. She pleaded: "Christopher tell them I am okay, and I can go to the bathroom, wash and clean myself and make my own meals, while you and Kevin do my shopping. Please Christopher?"

I looked up at Grandma and with a heavy heart I shook my head, fighting to hold back the tears before replying: "Grandma you have hardly done anything for two years. You do need the help this lady is offering you. I stood up and turned towards the door to walk out of the room, hoping she wouldn't see me cry. The next thing I heard was her shouting, "You all just want me in a home so you can sell my house!"

Things between me and Grandma were different from that day. It felt like I had betrayed her trust and she hated me for it, though deep down I knew she loved me. I was only doing what I thought best for her. She couldn't look after herself anymore. It was becoming too unsafe for Grandma to stay at home and I was not sleeping or eating due to the need to watch over her twenty-four hours a day.

My life already felt like I was cursed with my health, heartbreak and pain, but just when you think things can't get any worse...

Not long after Grandma had been placed in the care home, Kevin and the family put her house up for sale. The home which I was still living in. When I asked Kevin what would happen if the house sold quickly, he just shrugged his shoulders. I told him I would be made homeless. His lack of response spoke loud and clear. I was good enough to live there while I was looking after Grandma, but now I'm not needed he couldn't care less for my well-being. Within six months he had emptied the house. I understood it needed to be sold to cover the cost of the care home. The thing that hurt more was the way I was treated. I was practically left with nothing. All I had was a fold-up bed and a television, which was built-in thankfully. Kevin sold all the white goods, so I had no washer, dryer, fridge or freezer. There was no wardrobe or drawers. I had no choice but to come back to Wrexham because in a sense there was nothing left for me in Manchester anymore.

It felt like I was used by Kevin. He never asked me what I wanted or how I had been affected by Grandma's decline. Kevin has never really thought about how I felt about things. When I told Kevin that I would have to move back to Wrexham with Mum, he offered to drop me off. That was the most he had offered to help, though it felt more like it was to make sure I had gone. Off I went back to Mum's, temporarily.

Grandma sadly passed away suddenly, about a fortnight after I had moved back to Wrexham. I always beat myself up because I unfortunately never got the chance to hold her hand in her last precious moments.

I won't ever get that opportunity, but in my heart, I know she truly loved me and knew I did my best for her. Grandad would have been immensely proud of me for keeping my promise to him when he asked me to look after Grandma before he left. The commitment and support that I gave Grandma made us both close and far apart.

I miss her always, even though she tested my strength and patience every day. She scared the living hell out of me more times than I can remember, but I always feel blessed to have spent time with her and that I was able to help as much as I could, keeping that most important promise to Grandad.

Love you forever and always, Grandma!
Sleep peacefully,

Christopher xx

CHAPTER 23

Eczema and Sleeping Rough

I started having skin issues about twelve months before I came back to Wrexham. Originally it just was on my ears and face, constantly flaking like dandruff. It itched really badly and would peel off and become inflamed and sore. I visited numerous doctors. I was diagnosed with an eye infection and even a blocked ear. I was prescribed many types of antibiotics, ear and eye drops as well as steroid creams, but nothing seemed to work. I felt embarrassed and became very self-conscious. It even affected my socialising. I would make excuses for not going out. This then started to affect my confidence and self-esteem, especially when my personal hygiene became an issue because it was too painful to wash.

A couple of weeks after Grandma's funeral, I was given a written notice from Paul (Mums husband) which said I had three months to find somewhere to live, otherwise I would be homeless. I never expected this to happen, but once I came back from Manchester after the funeral, my eczema got worse. It got so bad that I had to go to Accident and Emergency for them to have a look at my skin. I wasn't sleeping. I was constantly in pain and my skin was weeping. It was red raw. I was told to cover it up and that there was nothing they could do for me. The hospital thought it could be down to my past health or stress levels.

When I got back the house Paul told me I couldn't live there any longer. He told me to go pack my stuff. He said pack a backpack with clothes and grab your medication. I felt so rejected and unloved at that time. I was as low as I could be.

The pain over my whole body was excruciating but that didn't matter to Paul. He just said he couldn't put up with my skin being everywhere. He said it was disgusting and dirty. He then drove me to the Council buildings to see a lady about homelessness. The lady explained my options. She offered me a place called a hostel, the same place that individuals released from prison go, or those fighting addiction. I explained to the lady that I couldn't go there with my health issues and medication, even though she understood she had nowhere else for me to go.

I contacted Jason (my cousin) while I was in the meeting at the council. Jason started laughing at me at first, thinking I was winding him up, until the lady spoke to him. He offered to put me up with himself and his daughter until I could get somewhere. When I walked out of the meeting, I thanked the lady for her advice.

Paul asked me where I was going and I replied that I was going to Jason's. As I started to walk towards the bus stop, Paul told me that I couldn't go to Jason's because he had a child. He then asked, "can't you pay for a Premier Inn or something?"

"Seriously?" I said, "anyone would think I'm loaded!" By the time I got to Jason's, all my cousins knew about my skin issues as Paul had told Laura, Jason's eldest sister. He also told everyone that it was contagious and I shouldn't be allowed in by anyone. This was total nonsense as no hospital or doctor had even mentioned it being contagious. Paul was being really weird and had turned nasty. Paul was always jealous of the relationship between Mum and me, though it seemed he had won this time as I had fallen out with Mum over this incident. I felt she didn't have my back. I lacked trust in everyone. If you can't rely on your parents, then who can you rely on?

The day after all this I had a meeting with Julie, my transplant co-ordinator, Dr Robertson, my transplant consultant, and Caron, my social worker. They were all shocked at how bad my skin was. My consultant was straight on the phone to a dermatologist to see what was recommended and to get me an emergency appointment. The doctor explained they needed to cover it up and take swabs. They would also need to take some blood cultures. The dermatologist asked if I would mind waiting around as he was in another hospital doing a clinic and would get to me in a few hours. I readily agreed. Julie then bandaged my legs up. I looked like a mummy. Julie commented that I was ready for Halloween a few months early. Julie knows that I would usually laugh at a comment like that. Instead, she could see my pain. Once I had most of my body covered to limit the chance of infection, I went to speak with Caron about my housing situation, my health and mental well-being.

Once I had shut the door to her office, I just broke down sobbing. I couldn't take anymore. I felt that I had no one I could trust and had lost all respect in my parents. My body felt like I had been burnt from head to toe, with excruciating pain and discomfort that never let up. I couldn't even sleep properly. It felt like one thing after another. Then, on top of all this pain and suffering, I was homeless. Sleeping on a sofa at my cousin's was never meant to be a long-term thing. My mental health was very much in tatters after all the trauma with Kevin and Grandma. I just didn't care about anything anymore. In all seriousness, I just didn't want to carry on battling. I had given up on life. What do I realistically have to live for?

Caron managed to talk to me and calm me down, reassuring me that things would get better. She offered to make a plan of action. In total honestly, I looked up at Caron thinking she was only saying that because it was her job, though I knew she always made me feel more like a close friend. I just didn't believe what she was saying. I had nothing else to lose. The plan of action we discussed was to first and foremost make sure that my transplant stays viable, then to sort out my skin issue and find a treatment that works. She then planned to arrange for me to see a psychologist about my anxiety and depression. "Talking to someone may help you," she said. After that the plan was to sort suitable accommodation near Jason and my cousins so that I had help with my day-to-day life close by. Once she had managed to calm me down and we had worked on a plan of action I began to feel a little better. Sometimes it's the simple things that make such a difference. Just having someone to listen to me helps more than that person could realise.

Before I knew it, Julie had popped into the office to tell me that the dermatologist had arrived. I picked up the cup of tea that Caron had kindly fixed me and took it with me. As I picked up my cup, Julie noticed that I was shaking a lot. She interjected, "I'd best carry that, otherwise I will need house-keeping to mop the floors after you!" I asked them where I needed to go. Julie showed me to a side room and in came the dermatologist. He undid all of Julie's exceptionally high standard bandage work. He explained that my eczema was extremely inflamed and raw. It was the most extreme case of eczema that he had seen.

I spoke with Dr Robertson about my previous and current health conditions, plus the downward spiral of bad news suffered recently. All that, mixed with the levels of anxiety and depression experienced in these extreme conditions, will cause any type of skin complications to flare up. With my immune system having to work overtime, my body can't recover as quickly as a healthy person's would. The doctor wrote up a routine of antibiotics, steroid creams and personal hygiene care. He then said to give it four weeks and then come back and see him. If it got worse, he said not to hesitate to ask the Renal Team for an earlier appointment.

I was living with Jason for around 14 months before I was offered a one-bedroom ground floor flat literally around the corner from him. This was ideal, but was this the break I needed from all the heartache of last few years?

Mum was still adamant that Paul had not kicked me out. She even had the audacity to say that I was the one who had blown it all out of proportion. Well, believe what you want, Mum, but you weren't there. What do you call being told I'm no longer welcome in his home and that I should grab my bags so that he can take me to the Council about somewhere to sleep from tonight? If that isn't kicking someone out I don't know what is? Mum carried on defending him and believed whatever came out of his mouth, because he can never do anything wrong. I just know that I won't ever set foot in his home again.

I will, of course, always love my Mum, but I have had to learn that I can't trust the closest of family members, the very ones I should be able to depend on. First my father made me homeless after Grandma's house was sold, and now Paul has done the same, and my Mum was standing by him. I am now left to face the world alone, bottling up all the dark and dreaded feelings that fill my head at night, preventing me from sleep and calm. Not allowing my body time to repair itself as I rest.

The world can be a lonely place when dealing with chronic health conditions and disabilities, though we are the people that get laughed at in the street or get left to fade into the background. We rely on the kindness and sincerity of family and friends, and yet here I am ALONE.

CHAPTER 24
Glyndŵr and Me

A few weeks passed, and during a meeting, when I was feeling low with anxiety and depression, my consultant was concerned about my health and well-being. Dr Robertson asked Caron to see if she knew of any activities, programmes or groups that I might be interested in. After such a turbulent few years, Caron thought that I should get myself a new focus and join a group or society where I could share my knowledge and wisdom to help others. I laughed at her at first and said, "what can I teach others?" But Caron always had a way of talking me round, getting me to give things a shot. Caron asked me to leave it with her to do some research and she would see what was available that I could easily access.

After only a short week or so Caron called me and asked if I fancied trying out a programme at Glyndŵr University, totally voluntarily. It was only one day a week, to help Social Work students understand the different lives and experiences of individuals who have been part of the Social Care services. She assured me that if I did not enjoy it then that would be totally fine and acceptable. I could just go the once and see. She also offered to come with me the first time for support, which I agreed to. I was immensely grateful.

Caron told me that she was going to introduce me to Liz, the Senior Lecturer in Social Care at Glyndŵr University. Liz convenes a group called Outside In, which is a focus group of individuals with expertise, through life experience, of using health and social care services. The group supports teaching and learning for the BA Hons Social Work and other degree programmes at Wrexham Glyndŵr University.

Social Work students and Outside In participation group: Year 1 - beginning September 2019

Session 1

I was excited but anxious as I didn't know what to expect. Caron came along, as she had promised, for moral support and introduced me to Liz, the programme leader. Liz was very friendly and tried putting me at ease. They were both extremely supportive in making me feel welcome. In the first session we introduced ourselves by writing our names down on a folded piece of card and explaining anything related to it. For instance, I remember someone saying her name was Kia and that she was named after the car her father liked. It was daft but we found it a good ice breaker. It was nice because it was the students' first day too, so everyone was feeling apprehensive and nervous. After the first hour the class was given fifteen minutes to grab a coffee or loo break. When we came back, the class was divided into small groups. The first group I joined consisted of Felicity (Fliss), Iola, Caroline and Bee.

When the students left, Caron and Liz asked me how I felt. I really enjoyed it. The students seemed to want to know me and everyone did what they could to make me feel comfortable. Liz then asked if I would come back next week. I said yes without really thinking about it. I thought to myself I could always ring Caron and cancel if I changed my mind.

Session 2

The second week I was feeling more optimistic. I arrived on my own this time and met with the other Outside In members in the café, where Liz came to chat with us a little before the session started. She explained that this lesson was more of a lecture style session. She said that we might find it a little boring because not all of it would be relevant for the Outside In members. The students I had met the previous week ushered me in to sit at their table, which was nice. They even remembered my name. Even though I was still extremely shy and quiet they did what they could to make me feel comfortable.

When I got home, I felt a little more settled and that I was doing something good. I enjoy learning and helping others, yet this did not feel too heavy or arduous. I began to feel that I belonged with this group. Everyone said hello as they walked past me at the table.

Session 3

This session was fun and interesting. I was feeling more comfortable and I joined the same group of lovely ladies who I had sat with the previous weeks. We were making a poster and getting to know each other a little more. The poster was to include all the things we liked, for example, football, wine, positive quotes, food and other things that we could all relate to. This showed that, regardless of our differences, we also had many similarities. The group was lovely, even if I didn't really get a word in. It was nice to feel part of something. In turn the ladies asked me a few questions and included me in the group task. Despite them telling me about themselves, I wasn't completely comfortable talking about myself just yet.

Session 4

Day trip to Liverpool visiting the Slavery Museum and looking at the beginnings of social work. The trip was to be not just a fun day out but a team-building exercise. The visit to the

Slavery Museum was interesting. Half the group met at the university and went on the train together, while the other half made their own way there. I got to know Iola, Fliss, Caroline and Rhi more during the Museum tour and on the journey back. There was also the Titanic section of the Museum. I felt the museums were definitely worth the visit. Lunchtime was nice and relaxed, well, until a cheeky seagull took a chance and decided to attack Iola's sandwich. This was definitely something that needed to be added to the next safety protocol for Liz! We were all laughing about it on the trip back to Wrexham. The second part of the day was a nice walk around the Albert Docks. David, another of the lecturers who went on the trip, knew all about the history of the dock and how it linked to the Social Work course. Everyone had a great day. I was very tired though when I got home.

Session 5

Unfortunately, I missed this session due to illness. Story of my life.

Session 6

I missed the previous week after becoming extremely run down and exhausted from my eczema playing up. This was making daily tasks, such as walking and getting dressed, difficult, never mind getting into university. I found out while I was in hospital that my eczema had become infected and caused me to become poorly.

Session 7

Today I was nervous about who I would be working with for my first group assignment. Liz had arranged the groups and hoped that everyone would get some value from the experience. The group had a few weeks to collectively produce a presentation to share with the rest of the class. When Liz read out my name, I took a deep breath. She then went on to read out the other names, which were four lovely ladies.

The new group consisted of Rhi, Hannah, Hayley and Bee. They all got on great, laughing and joking with each other. They included me, though I was happy to sit back and listen to them. I sat there with my hand on my head thinking, "Oh no! What have I got myself into?" I was glad they were talking the way they were. They discussed things they had got wrong, or different bad things that had happened to them, or things that made them laugh. They made feel so relaxed. We are all very similar: most in the group had had medical problems or involvement with Social Care services. This made me feel at ease. We were put into our groups to find out our strengths and similarities. Shockingly, I thought to myself we had many.

Bee, who had become the natural leader of the group, suggested that we make a WhatsApp group for us all to stay in touch while working on our project.

At the end of the session, Liz checked in on me to make sure I was ok. I was beginning to really find my place in the group and the class. I was thankful to Caron for literally saving my life as before starting University I didn't have anything to look forward to.

Session 8

Gosh! These ladies can talk! The group I was assigned to got together again, this time we were in more of a study-room to discuss the assignment. The discussions were very strong and we kept confidentiality at the forefront of our conversations, even in our WhatsApp group. I found WhatsApp very helpful as it took me a while to feel comfortable enough to explain my background.

I had told the ladies I was writing an autobiography about my life and health journey. They were very enthusiastic. They would constantly ask me to bring previews in for them to read. Liz would check in on how we were doing and ask if I was ok with the group. The group was fine, but, seriously, one man against four opinionated, talkative, passionate women? I was never going to get a word in. The ladies would disagree. I'm sure they would say I could give as good as I got. Ha-ha! Maybe they are right, but for now I have to pretend that I'm shy and innocent.

Session 9

Unfortunately, I missed this week yet again, due to my eczema. The ladies were fabulous at keeping in touch with me via our WhatsApp chats and videos. I was updated with everything. Bee even made sure that anything that was discussed was written up and made into work files. She printed one out for everyone each week so that we could add it to the portfolio, and we could refer back to it while writing up the assignment. Bee didn't know that I did not need to do an assignment and write it up, though it was nice to be treated with equal importance. I was grateful to the ladies for always checking in with me and not making decisions until I had been included.

Session 10

This was the final day to prepare the presentation for our first assignment. We decided as a group to come up with a video of our journey together, explaining our strengths, similarities and a quote we liked or disliked.

The final video had to consist of the following from each member.

- Strengths
- A picture to show the class whose story was being told
- A song reflecting that person's personality or battles

I also added a brief introduction to my life journey. The class members were shocked. A lot of them thought I was receiving support for mental health not physical health.

The video became our 'Car Share'. We were amazed at the final production, all credit to Rhi's media skills. We were excited but also very nervous about how the class, and most importantly the tutors, would react to our video.

Session 11

The day of the presentations was an anxious day filled with clammy hands and nervous tummies. You could feel the tension in the class as everyone worked on last minute adjustments. One by one each group stood at the front of the classroom. Each eye glued to the stories, feeling connected via each other's experiences and strengths.

As our group sat together awaiting our turn, my pulse felt like it was going to burst through my veins. I was wondering if we had got what the assignment was asking for. Did we fulfil the brief? It was too late to do anything about it now anyway. The time had come. It was our turn to present our video. Thankfully I didn't have to say anything about myself. I stood up there with the group members, glued to the screen. One by one our individual stories came on, with the class laughing at our pictures and singing along to our songs. Then, boom! Back to reality! My slide came on. My heart sank, my throat went dry, my mind thinking, "Shit! My story is out there now! My background for all to see. What will the class think?"

The only people who knew before were the four lovely ladies I worked with on the assignment. The end of the video came and all five of us must have been thinking, "thank fuck that's over!"

The applause from the class was more than any of us ever expected. There were even tears from members of the class. This gave me such a confidence boost to carry on allowing myself to build trust in others, especially these four crazy ladies.

CHAPTER 25

Covid-19 and Lockdown

Currently, as I sit here writing, I'm also experiencing the bonus of copious amounts of time to watch programmes on Disney Plus and Netflix. We are all in the middle of the coronavirus pandemic. I'm on day seven of the twelve weeks minimum self-isolation guidelines. Along with many millions of vulnerable people, I must adhere to the guidance as I'm in the extremely high-risk category, due to kidney transplants, immuno-suppressant medication and chronic kidney failure stage 4. I can really start to feel the frustration creeping in now, especially as I haven't been out or seen anyone for over a week. I am a sociable person and I struggle being on my own. I have far too much time to think. I know I have spent lots of time alone in hospital previously but there's always someone to have a quick chat with, or you can watch what's going on around you. The nurses and doctors were always saying 'hi' or teasing me. I have the added pressure of knowing this is just the beginning. At least eleven more weeks to go, if not a lot longer if I'm being realistic.

After sitting here day after day, I begin to think of all the negative, self-loathing thoughts I have had in the past, such as not being able to have children. In some ways that has been a good thing. My apologies to anyone reading this who is unable to conceive. After reading through the previous pages of this book, hopefully you have grown to love my way of thinking and even be able to laugh along with my twisted sense of humour - after all, that's what has got me this far.

The reasons I say I'm glad I couldn't have children lie in situations like this pandemic. I couldn't imagine having to be away from my child for a couple days never mind a minimum of twelve weeks. If I did have a family, I would have to self-isolate away from them. I wouldn't be able to witness their giggles while blowing bubbles at bath time, or even help with the home schooling. Well done to all those parents who are not only coping with isolation but also taking on a multitude of roles at this time. That to me sounds like hell. I would not be able to hold my child or help put them to bed. I think that fate works in mysterious ways. So perhaps for the first time in my life I'm happy not to have any children at home with me right now.

Liz, my tutor from Glyndŵr, has been emailing me often and staying connected, seeing how I am coping.

A health update during lockdown so far is that my eczema is under control, thankfully. This is also boosting my confidence and self-esteem. The clearer my skin is, the better the urostomy bags stick to my body, which means fewer leakages. Dialysis access has taken a few steps backwards, though this is a good sign as my kidney function has slightly improved. They have increased by 4% up to 18%, and the time period between blood tests has now stretched to every 6 weeks to try and limit my opportunities of contracting the Covid-19 virus.

Trying to keep focus and keep my brain active is already becoming a difficult task. So, I started on my second assignment last week. Unfortunately, I only had the opportunity to work with the second group (Holly, Rhi, Bee, Jess and Hayley P) in our class for just one session. It felt strange working with a whole new set of people.

April 2020

It's been a month now in lockdown.

I'm finding it hard being by myself. I have started to drift towards thinking negatively and have started to believe people may forget about me. I try to think of new ways to fill my day. I have never cleaned so much in my life! I tend to put music on and find a cupboard that needs a sort-out or a sink to give a good scrub.

It's getting difficult to stay positive currently. I'm really beginning to miss seeing Mum and speaking to her. We are normally so close, but she is working in a nursing home. She is also having to isolate herself from me. I have only seen her once, when she ferried me to and from getting my bloods taken. Mum has been doing my shopping. I transfer the money into her account, then text her a basic list. She then collects what she can, then calls me from the car so I can unlock the main entrance to the block of flats where I live. Mum then places the shopping in the hallway. I keep back at a reasonable distance, normally in the living room with the door closed so that we limit infection. Once she has placed the shopping in the hallway, she shouts through to me. Mum always shouts, "Love you!" before leaving. Then the door slams shut. Alone again in the small confines of my flat.

Then, with anti-bacterial wipes in hand I start to clean all the surfaces that Mum may have touched all the way to the shopping itself. I will then lock the door and put the shopping away. Wearing gloves, I wipe each item individually then place them in the correct cupboard or storage area. On Good Friday, Mum told me that as of Tuesday, she and Claire (my sister) would be going into total lockdown for 6 weeks as they are both working in the local care home. I was devastated, but, as usual, I just smiled and replied: "Ok Mum, I will be fine!"

Inside though, it felt like a knife stabbing into my heart. I get annoyed at myself that I'm unable to be honest with Mum and tell her how I truly feel. Mum explained that the earliest they would be able to come out of lockdown would be Sunday 25th May. They are both going to live at the care home to minimise the infection rate to the elderly.

All the time Mum was chatting away on the phone to me I was thinking some awful thoughts. I started regressing into a childhood state, thinking why would she do that when she has a son who needed her too? A dreaded thought also played like a scratched record. What if Mum or Claire got ill or, even worse, died? I can't bear thinking about it, but it was a recurring nightmare that played vividly in my thoughts.

Health update: the surgeon is planning future dialysis access and has decided to put a catheter into the side of my chest. This sounds dangerous but is a positive for me because it will be easier for me to connect myself, and is better for me to learn to do home dialysis when needed. This will give me as much independence as possible and allow me to carry on with university. I didn't like the thought of the original plans to either inject my arms or groin every day. The disadvantage of a fistula is infection control and possible clotting of the line.

June 2020

Currently lockdown has been extended until 17th August. As the rest of the country eases lockdown measures, my kidney function has gone down to 14%, only 4% away from putting in an access line for me to start dialysis. This is kind of scary, to think I am extremely ill, yet I don't feel it. I have been put onto a low phosphate and low potassium diet which I am finding hard to get used to. This diet literally restrains me from enjoying anything that I usually like. Just imagine denying your child a treat and watching their bottom lip quiver as they sulk. Yep! That is me, ha-ha!

Why is it when you're told you can't have something you crave it more? It's a nightmare. I know its sweets and treats that I can't have but I also have to limit carbohydrates and fat proteins. It's a full-time job working out the ingredients and all the do's and don'ts of this diet.

CHAPTER 26

Fears, Worries, and Nightmares

I don't think I could ever go through another relationship again while fighting for my life on dialysis for numerous reasons. My health will only get worse over time and my dialysis access is awful. I can't look after and protect someone knowing deep down inside that I can't look after myself. My biggest nightmare was my kidney transplant failing ever since I got it from Kevin, knowing that would be my last chance at a so-called normal life. I am currently living that nightmare, knowing it is failing plus the fact I will need dialysis through a line more than likely. Access via my arms and legs is not efficient enough for a graft or fistula. I am potentially a ticking time bomb, just doing everything physically, mentally and emotionally possible to keep positive. To make this transplant last until Christmas would be an amazing achievement. I can't thank Caron, Liz, Rhi and Bee enough for all their support, guidance and, of course, laughter during lockdown.

Bee asked me a question one evening when I was feeling low: "Why do you have nightmares? Is it because you fear dying?" It made me think, to be honest. I am afraid for the first time in my life because I know what to expect from dialysis and all the procedures necessary to ensure access.

No matter how many times I battle to keep myself going through health, mental, or social matters, someone will always stamp on my progress and make me feel vulnerable, weak and worthless. I am starting to wonder why I bother trying to make something of my life when people always destroy me.

Maybe it's a sign that I shouldn't be happy. I should be alone in lockdown with no family or friends. It does make me think: why have I battled for 30 odd years when I have nothing to show?

People keep asking if I would have another transplant if I could. In total honestly, I would refuse another. I have a few reasons why.

I don't think my body will take another major operation.

I think finding a match could be almost impossible.

Can I go through the thoughts and nightmares if it were to fail all over again?

I have had my fair share of chances in life. I don't deserve any more.

This is my biggest battle ever now, fighting to keep this kidney and stay off dialysis for as long as possible, but then when I need dialysis do everything in my power to stay alive.

I know I'm vulnerable, weak, scared, hurting and slowly dying inside, but somehow I always manage to say I am fine, with a smile waiting to help my friends and family. I always felt that if I showed I am struggling it would reveal that I am a failure and a coward, but I realize that not talking and opening up about your true feelings and worries can seriously cause you so issues with your self-esteem, mental health, and appearance. Most importantly it causes you to develop serious anxiety and depression. From my personal experiences with trust, respect and loyalty, I doubt everyone. With family, friends or even in a relationship, I am constantly doubting everything people say. I analyse everything. Sometimes I may come across to others as controlling as I need to know everything to put my mind at rest. I may come across as shy, ignorant, or rude, maybe even judgemental.

From my perspective, I would more than happily explain to anyone who has a question about anything. If I don't like the question, I simply won't answer.

But we do all need to talk more to help people combat mental health issues.

Final Words

I have a lot of issues that could eventually cause a massive chain of reactions over the next 18 months to 2 years. Lots of people keep telling me to stop thinking about what could happen next and basically wait and take each step as it comes, but I can't do that. I need to know each step of the process because, in my eyes, it's not just a case of waiting for my kidney function to reach 10% and then start my dialysis access, or whatever they decide is the best way forward. I also have to deal with the matter of when will I go on dialysis. I also want to learn to do it myself at home to give me a bit more independence. I am completely in the dark about this as I have always done it in a hospital unit, with the nurses doing all the priming and cleaning of the machine, as well as connecting and disconnecting me. All I did was turn up and sit there.

There is also the thought in my mind as to whether my home is efficient enough and suitable for me to dialyse in, or will I need to move, which, of course, comes with all the issues of moving.

I also live alone. What would happen if I was to become ill while I was on dialysis at home? There are still so many questions that I need reassurance on.

Loads of my family constantly say: "You will be fine! You have done dialysis for a decade, you will easily do it again." That is correct, but my access was shocking over a decade ago when I was last on it and it definitely ain't any better now! Some family and friends say: "Oh well, once you get another kidney transplant you will be back to your best!" Seriously, people! Getting a kidney isn't as easy as you think, and I know I am extremely fortunate to have had four by the age of 23! I know I am still relatively young, only being 34, and my nurses and friends would say I have a lot to live for.

I believe others deserve the chance to have this life saving surgery, I know mine hasn't been an easy ride, but I am still here fighting and hope to leave a long-lasting legacy. My message is that all individuals with chronic conditions have a voice. I know we don't have a degree, or a special title, but lecturers, social workers, students and medical practitioners learn more from patients than they ever will from reading textbooks.

Thank you once again for taking the time to walk with me along this journey.

I have poured my heart, soul and insecurities into every page, but I didn't want to beat around the bush and make out that things aren't as bad as most people believe. Chronic, hidden conditions don't make us any different in our hearts from the next person, so please don't stare at us like monsters, we can't help the way we move, look, or behave. All we want is to live as normal a life as you.

Take care, and I wish everyone all the best.

Chris.

Special Thanks Mum

Mum,

How do I even begin putting my thoughts into words?

I have tried to detail how I believe that you are the main reason I am still alive. I'm still here fighting for extra days, laughing at my jokes and yours. I'm still here winding you up and even being the root cause of your nightmares. However, I wouldn't be your brave boy, Chris, if I wasn't causing you mischief and mayhem. After all, that's my job. I wrote this book for you to hold my hand and retrace the steps we have taken to get to where we are today.

Take my hand at this time. I will support you and allow you to understand how my journey felt and looked to me. The number of times I suffered in silence and held my emotions in the pit of my tummy! I'm now allowing you to feel my pain, to see my hurt, to capture my smiles, but most of all to accept my gratitude for always being the one person that I could depend on. No matter what other struggles you were going through in your life, you were always there by my side and I know you will be for the rest of my life.

I'm going to take my emotional guard down and show my vulnerable side, which is not easy for me as you are already aware. I will try my best to explain. At this point I imagine you may need to get that fresh box of tissues, please don't get the pages wet, it took me years to write this (ha-ha)! I don't want you ruining the book.

It's my turn to wrap my arms around you and show you through my words why I love you, even if I don't often say it. Mum, it is truly felt.

We have always had an inseparable bond. I have never truly been able to open up and show my feelings, apart from my well-tried and tested emotions of anger and frustration. I believe it's thanks to your laid-back attitude that I was able to pull myself through the tough times.

People tell me I am an inspiration. I always laugh and think to myself that none of them have a clue what inspiration looks like. I saw the determination in your eyes, I felt the strength in your arms. I heard the conversations behind closed doors, and I heard your heart beating faster every time you held me close as a little boy.

Love you,

Christopher x

With Special Thanks – Bee

Special mention to the person who felt every emotion,

I would be honoured for you to have the heart and soul of my book; the paper copy I spent numerous hours on while in hospital or sat at home after uni. we instantly had a connection through the passion of making a change to people's lives who as we once are less fortunate but with true passion, determination, courage and will power. We both overcame our challenges and somehow by faith our paths led us to become such close friends. Maybe it is our Grandads watching over us, who knows? You from the very first day we met made me feel comfortable and welcoming with your warming smile. Working together on our first assignment was a right laugh and you made me feel a part of the team, gradually allowing me to open up in my own time. Working on my presentation with you was a nice challenge it opened your eyes to my world, which is not easy to talk about in front of a class but thanks to your determination and belief in my potential I did it.

I am honoured you can open to me and talk to me about anything, we made a promise at the beginning of the epidemic and I was in lockdown that we would always be there for each other no matter how things got.

Working on the book together was a master stoke it connected us, writing my life journey has been a hard-difficult process but it has also helped me to open up and express my true feelings and fears.

I can never truly thank you for all your support, guidance, laughs and the love you show.

We will make this book what we intended it to be through pure determination.

Will always be hear for you, Keep smiling.

Chris xx

With Special Thanks – Claire

Where do I start? The memories! Oh my God! The normal brother/sister relationships, the sibling rivalry, the arguing, fights, the tears shed, and the achievements and accomplishments.

Growing up, we were inseparable You were more like the protective big brother even though it was my job to protect you. You were the one who knew how to push my buttons: you knew exactly how to look at me or say something to wind me up.

Growing up, we were a formidable team, just me, you and Mum. Our bond was unbreakable, knowing Mum had our backs, fighting every battle alongside us, in our best interests. She would give up her last breath for us if she could, and we grew up knowing that. Mum would stand by us when we made our decisions, even the ones she knew would hurt us. Yet she let us learn for ourselves.

People say I'm inspirational because of what I have been through, but technically I didn't have a choice: this is just my life. You on the other hand had to deal with being palmed off to friends and family members like a ragdoll. You must've been thinking that you were being abandoned every time Mum had to take me to the hospital, sometimes for months at a time.

Both in our thirties now, we could never have imagined that. You supported me through the pain, separations, and heartbreaks. I want to tell you how much I really appreciated your time, your listening ear, and your advice, even if I did have to take it from my baby sister.

I want to show my love and appreciation and one day I may still get to see you settle down and get married. Hurry up though, as I would also like to be an uncle!

All jokes aside, Mum would love to be a Grandma and I'm unable to do that for her, so this one, Sis, is down to you. You might be a pain in the arse most of the time, but I wouldn't change a thing.

Here is the story you tell everyone you meet about me, so I will set the record straight and tell my version of it.

One day, Claire and I were arguing, and she wound me up so much that I threw a bottle opener straight through a square glass window door, while Claire was on the other side of it. She didn't get hurt, thankfully, but straight afterwards we cleaned it up like nothing had happened and went swimming with friends. I came home and Claire had gone to her Dad's after swimming and Mum went mad.

I told Mum Claire had done it and when she got home from her Dad's on Sunday, she got grounded for two weeks and lost her pocket money.

I felt bad afterwards and owned up to smashing the window. Mum went mad at me and grounded me for lying for one week (but I got to keep my pocket money. Ha-ha!).

Claire, I'm sorry. You have never dropped this and you bring it up all the time. We have learned to laugh at it now. I want you to imagine me saying:

"Thanks for all the fun!"

All my love, hugs and kisses, Claire, from your big, better, brother,

Chris xx

With Special Thanks – Mark

The first time we met was when Mum, Joe, Claire, and I moved into the army house in Radcliffe. You came over, all cheeky, as always, offering to help. We must have been around six or seven years old and we had just started Radcliffe County Junior School. We were never really friends in school because I was always playing football, or not in school due to my health.

Our friendship blossomed during our time at high school, me playing sports with Jason, and you chasing the girls. You are still as cheeky and always playing the clown, helping me to chase the ladies (sorry, Amanda, he loves you deep down).

In high school you always had my back, and especially when that dickhead lad punched me straight in the stomach during a lesson. The lesson turned into total chaos by the time it had finished. Everyone was looking for him and blocking exits. The next day all the lads got called to the hall and I was told that if I arranged a fight again, I would get expelled and all the boys were going wild, saying how that lad deserved a beating.

Then came college and girls, relationships, heartbreak. We have argued and fallen out, but never for too long. I have watched you grow from a boy to a bigger boy (okay gentleman … nah, that's too kind! We'll settle for 'man'. That's the best I'm going to stretch to. I was so proud of you when you got engaged and became a Daddy to three beautiful children,

Alex, Georgia, Chloe, and Aiden along with taking on Jessica and Connor, loving them as your own.

One of my proudest moments was becoming a godparent.

Your children make me laugh when we're chatting on-line and I hear them all through the headset, asking about me. It makes me laugh when they nick off with your headset and start telling me about things that have happened.

It's the cutest thing when I come over and they get excited.

Thank you for making my life fun. Thanks for fulfilling my dream of becoming a godparent. Thanks for your support, laughter, and advice.

We have been through so much. I hope there are many more years of laughter and fun to come.

Cheers,

Chris

With Special Thanks – Jason

Being the joker of the family and never taking life seriously, you always make me laugh and smile. You - the crazy loveable thug, born on my actual birth date, just a year later. We are cousins: however, in my eyes, you are more like the brother I never had. Some of my earliest memories are when we were toddlers arguing over toys.

We have grown older, but never dismiss the impact of all those hours you sat with me in the hospital. You caused mayhem when I was fit enough to get out of bed! You would play games with me and challenge me to things, but you would always win. Even when I was ill you would kick my ass, and nothing much has changed. We practically lived in each other's homes and even lived together for a spell.

I remember kicking a ball in the yard, or anywhere we could, to be honest. We were just two lads causing mischief, yet you always made sure I was living a fun life. Even if we were being stupid, you would make sure I was safe. We went to different primary schools but when we were at high school, we were inseparable.

The trouble we would get into, ordering kebabs and pizzas to the hospital ward while I was hooked up to the dialysis machine! Two teenagers winding up the nurses to the best of our ability. You got me through dialysis and made it more fun. You have seen me at my worst and still stood by me.

You have seen me when my body was failing. You have witnessed my highs and lows. You helped me through the heartbreak of my failed relationships. I'm so honoured to be able to sit here and witness you as a father of two beautiful daughters, Evie-Mai and Molly. You are a fantastic father and you're doing something I could only wish to do, that is, bringing another life into this world.

I wish you all the happiness and all the luck in the world. I can never express in words how grateful I am for your unrelenting support and kindness. I have tried my best to show my appreciation through my book and in life. I hope you understand the impact you have had on my life throughout my journey. Most of it fun, some of it scary but most of all you have shown me an unbreakable bond of brotherhood.

Cheers,

Chris

With Special Thanks – Caron (Social Worker)

I honestly don't know, how I can truly explain or show my gratitude towards you. In my eyes, you're an absolute diamond. You are such an influential person and so motivated to do the best you can for everyone. You go over and above fulfilling your job role. Your professionalism is exemplary, keeping to boundaries yet always exuding the rapport of a true friend with a heart of gold.

I believe that social workers should be able to build a friendly professional relationship with their service users, forging trust and empathy. A social worker should always use their communication skills to allow them to be able to read the body language of their service user and not need words
Caron, you have seen me through so many difficulties and heartbreak. You never allowed the struggles to consume your thoughts, you always managed to get me the amount of help that I needed and believed in my strength while fighting my battles alongside me. You have helped me build confidence and find my self-worth. Thanks to you I am slowly but surely becoming the gentleman I am today.

You are always there to listen, no matter how busy you are. I never get the sense that I am just another one on your caseload, or, after the 10th call of the day, that I am wanting too much of you. You never huff or puff or tell me that I need to figure it out alone. I know you are quietly walking my journey alongside me, encouraging my victories and buffering the difficulties. You give me a call to make sure I'm on track, making me feel valued and worthy of your time.

You make sure I have all the tools to cope, regardless of whether I'm in the hospital or at home.

My proudest moment was when you accompanied me to Glyndŵr. You sat in the audience like a proud parent willing me to do my best. You got to witness the strength I have harvested and the confidence that has been built in such a short time via attending Glyndŵr. You were beaming with pride. You were ever the professional, holding in the emotions, with your sidekick, Julie, by your side. I could tell that you were both on my side, fighting the battles with me, standing close by, ready to catch me if I fell, hoping I realised my potential to become an independent, confident gentleman. I hope I have proved to you that I can do this, and that's thanks to your support.

You looked so proud and pleased, more than I had ever seen you before. Your smile, as I entertained and educated the class with my presentation at Glyndŵr, really decorated your face. You even smiled when I mentioned you, even though I knew deep down you were possibly recoiling with embarrassment. To you, this is just doing your job. But to me, you are guiding me through my life and making it as painless as possible.

You honestly deserve some accolade for how amazing and committed you are towards your job. You are an inspiration to many budding social work students.

'Thank you' seems so insignificant for the effort and work you have put in over fifteen years and more. That is an achievement for which I count myself extremely lucky.

From the bottom of my heart, I want to say thanks for being amazing.

From Chris x

With Special Thanks – Julie (Renal Transplant Nurse)

Julie was one of the first nurses I ever met when I came to Wrexham. I have grown so close to her that she feels more like a second mother to me. Even though she is very professional, she always goes out of her way to make me laugh and feel comfortable. She would never allow me to see how busy she was, or if she was stressed. She would always show an interest in my personal life.

She would playfully question me about what I had been up to, and she would ask about any relationships I had on the go. She would make me out to be a Lothario. If I didn't have a girlfriend, she would say to me things like: "You don't need a woman, listen to your Mum", or "You have all us lovely nurses here running around after you. What more could you wish for?" Her personality is infectious and her smile intoxicating. You can't help but smile when she is around: she won't let you be sad for long. Every time I saw her, she would come over to me and give me a hug and smile and say, "Hello, gorgeous! Oh God, you smell nice!" These things help build my confidence bit by bit.

It has been a real pleasure and privilege to have you as my transplant nurse. You have supported me not only through my medical difficulties but also my relationships and breakups and the lowest points of my mental battles. You even stood by my side when I was having the transplant from my Dad. Now you are getting to see me at my personal best, even though my body is failing me yet again.

Please don't underestimate your worth and the help and support that you have given me throughout my life. You are truly inspirational and I'm sure your daughter is immensely proud of you, just as I am proud to have met you.

I just wanted to say a huge thanks from the bottom of my heart. I would say thanks to my kidneys but we both know how shit they are! I also know I could say thanks with diamonds, but I'm broke, LOL, so this dedication will have to do for now.

I told you I was writing a book - now you're getting to read it.

Keep smiling,

Chris x

With Special Thanks – Liz (Senior Lecturer in Social Care at Glyndŵr University)

The first time I was introduced to Liz was through Caron, who explained Liz would do anything she could to make me feel comfortable within the class at Glyndŵr. Liz was very welcoming, introducing herself and asking if we would like a coffee before meeting the other members of Outside In, who were also nervous before we all got introduced to the students. Week by week Liz would show respect and belief in my potential to help others. Always smiling and laughing, helping to create a warm friendly environment. At first when you would say my name in class I would think "oh no!" But over time, I realise you were building my confidence to speak about myself in front of everyone. When you praised me after my presentation, you told me how proud and privileged you felt to have me as part of your team. I will always be grateful for being asked to participate in Outside In and look forward to many years working together.

Thanks for your support, guidance, and most important, having faith in me.

Christopher x

Wrexham dialysis nurses,

To all the amazing lovely ladies who have become more like my second family always there supporting me through my toughest times as well as winding me up and making me see the funny side of dialysis.

Thank you all love Chris x

Thanks Gran,

Thank you for all your amazing support and laughs over the years, you are the living Mrs Brown with some of the things you come say and do.

Love you loads Christopher x

With Special Thanks - Dr Lewis (Pendlebury Hospital 1986 till 2002)

I truly owe this gentleman. In my eyes, and in the eyes of many thousands of babies, children and adolescents, he is the man who has made the difference to our lives. He never gave up on me when my parents were told I would be very unlikely to survive my first 24 hours. He Never supported me time after time, using all his medical knowledge and interventions, sometimes ones they weren't sure would help me, but he took that risk in order to keep me alive. I had the pleasure of seeing him back when I was around 23, not long after the 4th transplant. He was over the moon and proud to see me still battling on.

Thank you for never giving up on me.

Christopher

With Special Thanks – Dr Robertson

It feels like I have known you all my life. I'm not sure if that's a good thing or not! The first time I met you I think I was around 18-19 years old. I was so terrified of you and I knew you could tell. You were the first doctor I recall being straight to the point and who treated me with respect and understood I was an adult, which I technically was even though I didn't look it. My height always lets me down in this area, though I can sometimes get away with a cheaper bus ride (or a child's cinema ticket) if the conductors squint a little.

You have helped me to find the silver linings in all my issues. We have been through hell together, especially all the complications with dialysis access and my eczema, plus various infections. However, here we are fifteen years later, battling dialysis access issues again, trying to prepare me for the future. It has been one hell of a rollercoaster ride, but you did your risk assessments and buckled me in efficiently, sticking by me. You have witnessed me at my best and you have stood there alongside me at my worst.

Thank you for all your support, guidance and laughs.

Christopher

With Special Thanks –
Dr Glover

I can't actually recall the first time we met, which is obviously the sign of a good doctor. Those who just appear and do their thing unceasingly are rumoured to be at the top of their game. I have always looked up to your opinions and your advice has been gratefully received. You show such dedication to what you do, making the experiences of myself and other patients the best that they can be in the circumstances. You allow us the time to fully understand your planning process. You ensure your availability for questions and answers, affording us the time to understand why you're doing things in the way you have planned.

We have been through so many twists and turns through the years. You have always strived to do your utmost to support the difficult decisions, and be there to buffer the unforeseen outcomes and celebrate the more successful outcomes too. Your support has been much appreciated.

Thanks for your support and guidance.

Christopher

With Special Thanks –
Dr Thomas

Thank you for all your support and guidance and for being your normal crazy self, striving to make me laugh in the most difficult of times. I can recall when you came under Dr Robertson's wing while you were training. I am honoured we were given the opportunity to have 'grown up' together. Well, the years have passed but I didn't grow in height, more in tenacity over the years. You, however, grew in knowledge, understanding, and empathy even your jokes only got a little better. Keep working on that bedside manner! Things have changed so much that you are now one of my main consultants.

Congratulations on bagging yourself such an accolade as to have me on your patient list. Things worked out ok in the end!

Keep doing what you do best, brightening up the day, and saving as many people as possible. I just wanted to give you a mention in my book, so I thought this was the best way, after all, you have heard me mention it enough over the years.

Thanks for being great.

From Christopher

With Special Thanks – Nick, Social Work Tutor at Glyndŵr University

Thank you, Nick, for your support, and for your willingness to help include me in all outside meetings and any projects or ideas you had. Your ideas make learning more creative and practical, not only for the students but also for Outside In members as well. Unfortunately, due to lockdown we haven't been able to work together as much as we would have liked.

I think your way of making the degree course not just academic, but also more related to real-life situations will definitely help the students.

Once again, your support has been amazing.

Take care

Chris

With Special Thanks – Outside In

Thank you to all the lovely individuals who have helped me understand the important role of this part of the Social Work degree. This has taught me and the students about how Social Services have impacted upon your lives. You were all like parents looking out for me and you allowed me to grow into the group until I felt comfortable to express my experiences.

Gayle, you always gave me so much advice.

Eluned, your paintings opened my eyes to a different way of communicating.

Jenny, your presentation was interesting and opened my eyes to the conflicts people face.

Steve, what can I say, a true gentleman.

Sylvia, the boss in my eyes, but so down to earth and funny.

Sandra, always a laugh and full of advice, like Gayle.

Graham, loved your poem and presentation.

Tim, always full of advice and a pleasure to meet you.

Darren, full of knowledge but we didn't see each other much, hope you're feeling better.

Hope, an absolute pleasure to meet you and Angel.

Jade, such a young ambitious lady with a powerful background.

Keep doing the amazing work you all do and hope to see you all in uni again one day

Take care,

Chris

With Special Thanks – Students Group 2019-2021

Thank you to all the lovey ladies and, of course, Rob and Phil. Outside In and being involved with this programme has not been easy, but it has helped me with my confidence via opening up to a class about my background and my struggles. One major thing I learnt from this was that I can never change my past, but I can use it to shape my future and help people like yourselves to understand the impacts.

Thanks for being by my side. Even when I wanted to quit you never gave up on me.

Take care

Chris

Milton Keynes UK
Ingram Content Group UK Ltd.
UKHW011950110823
426759UK00012B/181/J